CW01064487

Ketogenic Diet

And

Intermittent Fasting

(2 books in 1)

Keto For Woman & Keto And Intermittent Fasting

The ultimate beginners guide to know your food needs with a low-carb diet for a perfect mind-body balance and understand the Metabolic Autophagy to Activate the Anti-Aging Process

By

Kyndra Backer

TABLE OF CONTENTS
KETO FOR WOMEN

TABLE OF CONTENTS
KETO AND INTERMITTENT FASTING

Keto For Women

The ultimate beginners guide to know your food needs, weight loss, diabetes prevention and boundless energy with high-fat ketogenic diet recipes

By

Kyndra Backer

INTRODCTION

Congratulations on purchasing Keto for women: The ultimate beginners guide to know your food needs, weight loss, diabetes prevention and boundless energy with high-fat ketogenic diet recipes and thank you for doing so.

The following chapters will provide you all the necessary information, facts and scientific explanations that you need to know and master the keto diet. You will find the details explanation on what is the keto diet based on, what are the ketones, what happens in your body when you go keto, how the ketogenic diet will heal and improve many of the processes and organs of your body, how the ketogenic diet is pretty good for people who suffer from diabetes, polycystic ovaries syndrome, seizures, and Alzheimer, the special benefits of the ketogenic diet on women, how it reduces and prevents age-related conditions and many other important and interesting information.

If you came here it is because you are interested in changing your feeding plans, your habits, your body, your lifestyle, and many other things. Let us tell you that you came to the right place. We want to warn you that this might be a difficult process, some of the things written here may not work equally for you than it did for someone else, so we want to ask you to go and see a specialist before making any change to your alimentation

There are plenty of books on this subject on the market, thanks again for choosing this one! Every effort was made to ensure it is full of as much useful information as possible, please enjoy it!

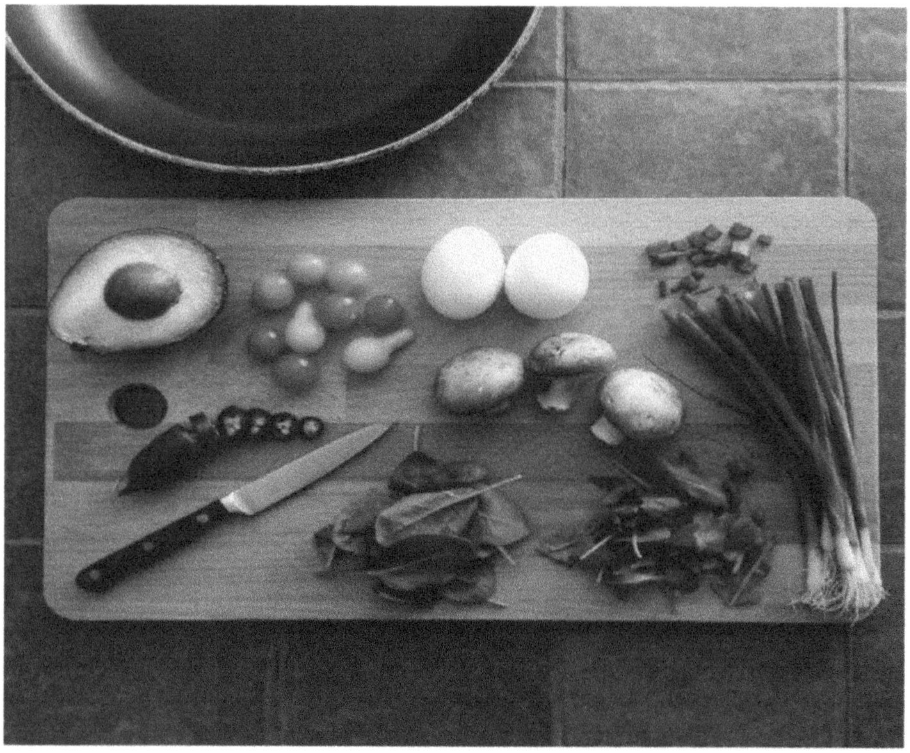

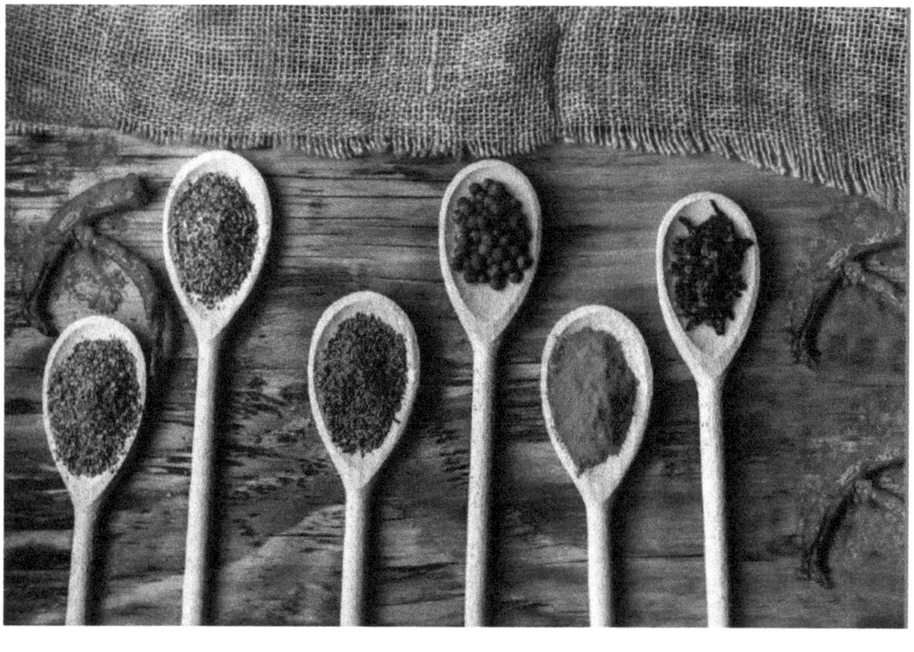

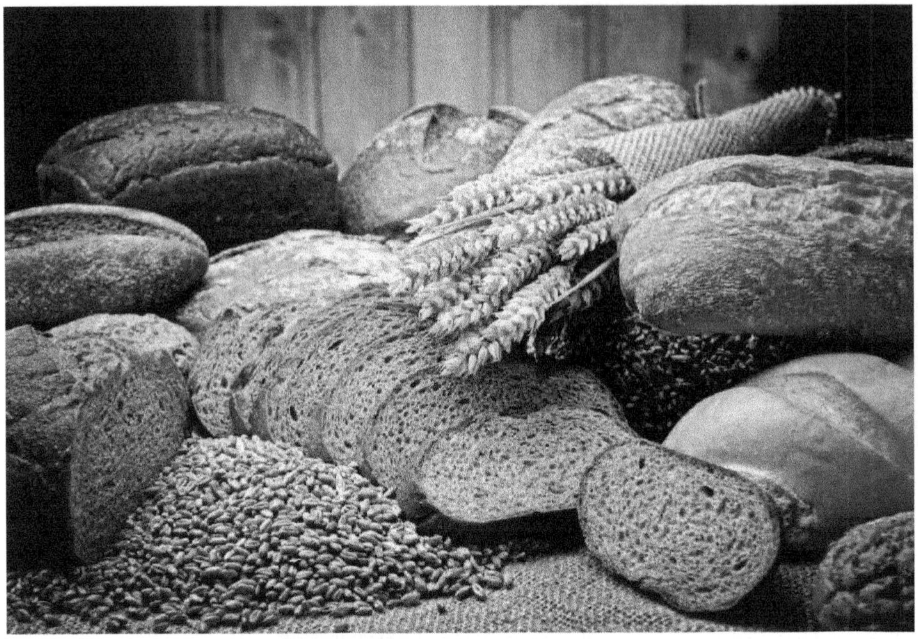

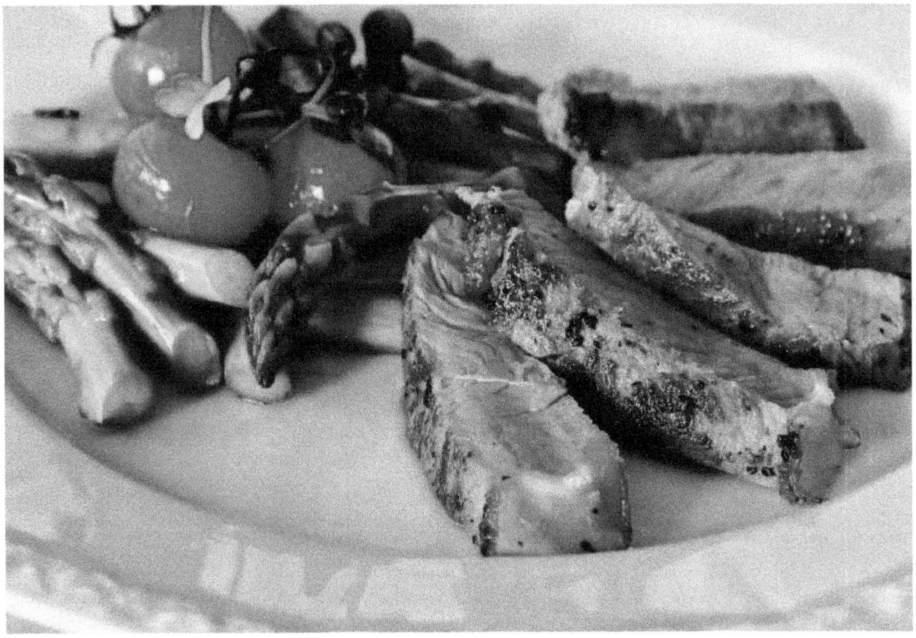

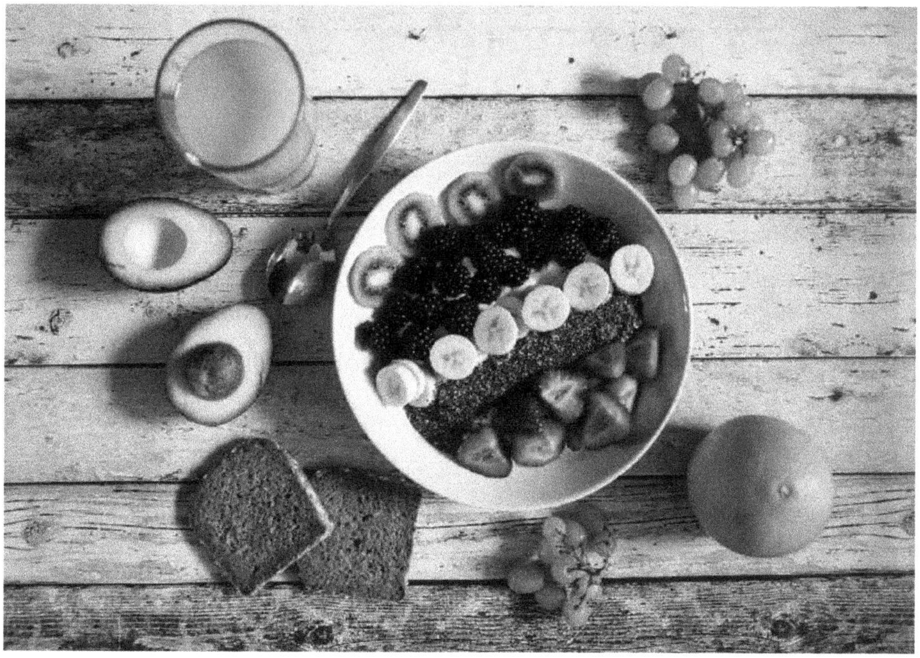

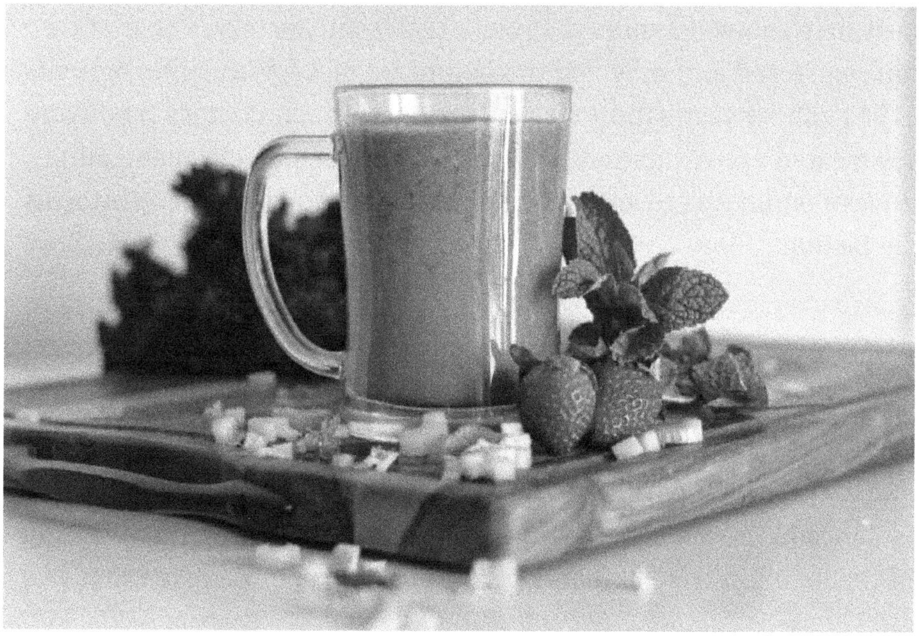

CHAPTER 1:
WHAT IS THE KETOGENIC DIET?

The Keto or ketogenic diet consists mainly of the ingestion of 75% fats, 20% high-value biological protein and 5% low glycemic index carbohydrates. That percentage should be applied to every meal. People who want to start with this diet must understand that this is not a diet, but this is a whole new lifestyle and it should be taken as it.

We want to mention that this type of diet has years in the market and has been subject of research on many occasions, demonstrating, in all cases, the wonderful benefits it has on health. This feeding plan is not only for adults; children and teenagers could also use it; so it is highly recommended.

The Keto diet has its beginnings near the 1920s and was made specially as a treatment for the people who suffered from seizures. Over time, and after a lot of researches and studies, the diet surprisingly showed results that were really satisfactory. The first case that possibly has been registered and in which the ketogenic diet for epileptic patients was applied was in 1911. The investigation was led by two French doctors who were Gulep and Marie. They treated approximately 20 persons, between children and adults. The objective of the investigation was to apply this type of diet, added to other protocols known as intermittent fasting.

The ketogenic diet is also very popularly known to lose weight, and lower blood sugar levels considerably, but it is important to know that sugar, gluten and other components that are not within the food permitted in this diet or method of ketogenic nutrition must be eliminated.

As we mentioned above, the major part of the food that we are going to consume is healthy fats, such as avocado, bacon, and peanuts, to mention some of them. In the following chapters of this book, you will be able to see some recipes or plans that you can apply in this diet.

The objective we want to achieve applying the keto diet is to reach a metabolic state in which ketones are the primary energy source of our body. This is achieved by following the diet regularly, with commitment and discipline.

This diet is not based on dietary restrictions, but on significant changes in lifestyle and eating habits, in which we are going to eliminate from our menu processed foods based on refined flours, sugar, and soft drinks. It is a diet that manages to heal marvelously and allow adequate cellular regeneration; Therefore, it improves and even eliminates some diseases, if applied in an evaluated manner with a specialist.

And these changes in the organism are due to the fact that this feeding method gives us the adequate tools for the best functioning of the cellular environment on our organism, and it does so by providing amino acids, essential fats for our body, vitamins, and minerals. This diet is amazing since it doesn't just allow you to lose weight but also makes you feel energy levels that you haven't before.

Any diet can be ketogenic if their bases are respected and if we have the knowledge of cellular processes and metabolism. Diets that can be considered ketogenic are those that force our body to use fats as a source of energy. Fasting can be considered ketogenical since by spending so many hours without eating, the body runs out of glucose and start to use ketones instead. Known this, we can say that a diet in which the lack of carbohydrates is replaced with other foods that has high contents of nutrients can be a ketogenic diet

The main objective of the ketogenic diet is to make our body to get into ketosis, lowering or decreasing to only 5% the intake of carbohydrates. This is a diet low in carbohydrates, and rich in fats that have been compared several times with the Atkins diet and other low-carbohydrate diets, so we share the idea that any diet where these percentages of food are distributed in similar amounts are ketogenic diets, or as it is abbreviated keto diets.

When we start with the ketogenic diet, we decrease the consumption of carbohydrates and replace them with healthy fats. Once this is done, the body will reach or get into a metabolic state called ketosis. In this state, the body is going to become incredibly efficient, transforming the fats in our body into energy. This process will also convert the accumulated fat in our body into ketones, hence supplying the brain with more energy. It should be noted that this eating plan generates higher energy levels than the ones generated by the usual feeding methods.

There are some foods that should be avoided when we are implementing this diet; Some of them are the following:

- Foods with high levels of sugar such as soft drinks, candies, fruit juices, cakes (in this case we would be talking about cakes made with refined flour), and other sweets.
- Foods that are derived from wheat like rice, pasta, cereals or starches.
- Some fruits should be eliminated due to their high amount of sugars. The only fruits that will be allowed are small proportions of forest fruits such as strawberries, blackberries, kiwi.

- The vegetables or legumes. Within this classification are: sweet potatoes, carrots, cassava, among others
- Lentils, chickpeas, beans or legumes.
- Some types of sauces. We would have to evaluate their preparation, as well as the condiments to use. In the keto diet, it is widely recommended to use natural condiments and sea salt mainly.
- Saturated fats are eliminated from this plan. The intake of refined oils, like margarine, mayonnaise, etc. is restricted or limited.
- Alcohol consumption is reduced. As it has high sugar and carbohydrate content. There are some drinks that are allowed in regulated portions and in small quantities.
- The dietetic foods are eliminated preferably; since in their majority and according to several studies, they have a high content of sugar. We recommend that you read very well the labels of the products that you are consuming, as the majority of these dietetic products are more harmful than the regular ones.

Similarly, there are many foods that can be consumed in the keto diet, most of these foods have a high content of nutrients and vitamins that restore the proper functioning of each of our organs.

As you enter this world, you will know which types of food can help you and bring certain benefits to specific organs. For example, a vegetable that is widely consumed in the keto diet is spinach. This vegetable has a high magnesium content that helps, among other things, to eliminate fatigue and it is a vital food for the brain. Just like the spinach, there are many other superfoods that, if applying this system of conscious feeding, you will get to know gradually.

Among the foods that we can consume are the following:

- The vegetables low in carbohydrates. Preferably it is recommended to consume in higher proportions green vegetables, but you can also eat onion, green onion, tomato, bell peppers, and others
- Fish. Such as salmon, tuna, sea bass, and a wide range of fish.
- Meats are also allowed either red meat, ham, bacon, chops, pork, etc..
- Eggs are widely allowed.
- Butter and creams are allowed, preferably those made with organic materials or milk from grass-fed animals are recommended.
- Cheeses are also allowed. However, the cheeses that are processed are suppressed, by which it is recommended to consume mozzarella cheese, goat cheese, blue cheese, etc...

- Healthy oils such as extra virgin olive oil and coconut oil are very commonly used as well as avocado oil.
- The condiments made naturally. Preferably it is recommended to use sea salt and Himalayan salt, also to season with green natural vegetables like green onion, and coriander, for example.
- It is advisable to consume water. In any feeding plan, the consumption of water is required for the good functioning of the intestine, and the organism in general.
- Last but not least, nuts. They must be consumed in a moderate way. The nuts that you can eat are flax seeds, almonds, walnuts, pumpkin seeds, and chia seeds.

As you have been able to observe, the ketogenic diet is strict and must be followed carefully if you want your metabolism to enter into ketosis. When this food plan is used to eliminate a disease or improve the health of a patient it is necessary to follow it strictly and rigorously so that the body can feed on energy from ketones.

Perhaps, the first few days will be complicated, but once you go through the process called keto-adaptation, you will see the wonderful benefits of practicing this diet, where you will not feel in any way the need to consume processed products, in fact, there are reports and studies that indicate that a person who reaches ketosis can fast intermittently or not with great ease because he has an inexhaustible source of energy due to the ketones produced.

The ketones as you will see in the next chapter, are an inexhaustible source of energy for the whole organism and in greater proportion for the brain. All of our organs consume a certain amount of energy, when we eat, we do not eat to provide calories to our body, but to provide energy to our organs so that each one of them can continue working correctly. And that is exactly what we want to achieve when we feed ourselves ketogenically.

CHAPTER 2: WHAT ARE KETONES?

This is a concept that comes from the organic chemistry that is seen in high school. It is an organic compound, formed by a group of carbonyls attached to two carbon atoms. The first thing we are going to do is define what a carbonyl functional group is. It consists of a carbon atom that connects, so to speak, with a double bond to an oxygen atom. This type of group is obtained in soda water or blood, as you will expect. The same one is connected with two organic radicals, therefore, we can say that two free bonds are connected to the carbonyl group. These chemical connections are the ones that allow us to differentiate carboxylic acids from aldehydes, alcohols, and ethers. Ketones can be considered less reactive than aldehydes and other organic compounds.

As previously explained, ketones have a similar structure to aldehydes, since both have the carbonyl group. However, the biggest difference between them is that they contain two organic groups instead of hydrogens.

As expected, there are different types of ketones, which are divided according to:

- The structure of their chain: They can be differentiated by the structure of the chain, they can be aliphatic, because the two organic groups that are connected with their carbonyl group, have the structure of the alkyl.
- The symmetry of their radicals: This classification is used when studying the radicals, which are connected to the carbonyl group. When they are the same, as you would expect, can be called symmetrical ketones, but in the case that both are different, they are called asymmetrical, being these the most common in chemistry.
- The saturation of its radicals: Finally, another method of classification. It will depend on the saturation of its carbon chains; if they have the structure of alkenes, the ketone will be unsaturated, on the other hand, if they have the structure of alkanes, it will be called saturated ketone.

There is another type of ketone but is not characterized by any of the three previous classifications. These are called diketones because they have within their chains, two carbonyl groups in their structure. As we mentioned above, these groups are the connection of a carbon atom with an oxygen, connected by two covalent bonds.

Now, to get a little deeper into this subject, let's take a look at some properties of ketones, both chemical and physical:

Physical: Mainly, we can observe that the boiling point of these substances is much lower than alcohol's and have the same molecular weight. As for aldehydes, they do not have a big difference in their boiling point, but both have the same molecular weight.

On the other hand, ketones are soluble in water, but as the chain becomes more complex, solubility decreases.

Regarding the smell, ketones that have a small size, have a pleasant smell, medium size has a strong and unpleasant smell. Finally, the bigger ketones are odorless.

The physical state will depend on the number of carbon they possess since ketones with less than ten carbons are liquid, but those with more are solid.

Chemical: In this case, we have many more properties than in the physical ones. They are:

- Its acidity. Thanks to its carbonyl group, ketones are acid.
- Another noticeable characteristic of the ketones is their reactivity. Ketones are widely used as a product that can synthesize other compounds. For this reason, ketones can be used to make the addition of alcohol, producing hemiacetals, which are not very stable. Another addition that can be made is with ammonia and some of its derivatives, forming a group of substances called imines, which are also chemically unstable.
- They are less reactive than aldehydes.
- Ketones are difficult to oxidize and this can only be achieved with strong elements such as potassium, to say one, thus producing an acid.

Now that we have explained what a ketone is and some of its properties, we can start the book as it should be done.

As you can imagine, ketones are widely used both in industry and in everyday life. We can often find them in perfumes and paints since they are responsible for stabilizing these compounds. Sometimes they serve as preservatives because they do not allow some components of the mixture to degrade quickly. Ketones can also be used as solvents for paints and textiles, in addition to this, they are used in the pharmaceutical industry as well as in those factories that manufacture explosives.

The first thing we must ask ourselves is where to find them in nature. They are found in a lot of places such as human cortisol hormones, testosterone, progesterone, fructose, among others.

It has been proven that some ketones are found in natural sugars in really small amounts, they are found in the fructose, being it a type of sugar. The cells found on the fructose are called ketoses, which can be found on fruits and honey. Although they are ketones, the consumption of them is not recommended for the ketogenic regime, since the concentration of ketones is so small that we will not get benefit of them.

One of the functions that can be done by ketones is the biosynthesis of fatty acids; being this the purpose of the book. What is wanted with this diet is that, through ketosis, a better burning of fats is achieved. In this case, these ketones are generated due to the excessive production of the acetic enzyme. Then, the process of generating the ketone is activated, thus making the cell spread throughout the body thanks to the circulation and goes to the vital organs, such as kidney, muscles or even the brain.

But talking specifically of ketones and what they can do inside our bodies is shocking. The first thing that is done is to release the ketones when the body takes fats instead of carbohydrates as a source of energy. This manages to burn a large amount of fat. That is one of the reasons why in some diets is preferred the consumption of fat than carbohydrates. But, what does this generates?

Levels of glucose in the blood are reduced because carbohydrates become sugar for our body.

In our body, ketones have the function of burning fat to generate energy. For that reason, we recommend diets high in fats and low in carbohydrates; to force our body to generate ketones capable of generating energy. Because in the case that there is a high consumption of carbohydrates, the body will be forced to generate energy through glucose.

Since you know that ketones are cells that you need in your body, you should also guess that there should be a normal or average amount of such cells. By this, we mean that there is a level of ketones in our body which is considered "normal", as is done with other cells, such as white blood cells for example.

Therefore, among the levels of ketones in the blood, are the following:

1. Less than 0.5 mmol/L: this means that there are normal levels in the blood. This level corresponds to people who have a diet that fits in normal, regarding the consumption of carbohydrates, fats, lactic, etc.. But what does this mean? Well, that the main source of energy of these people is fructose, or better said, carbohydrates, which implies that fat is not being burned, or not thanks to ketones.
2. The ketone's level in blood between 0.5 and 1.5 mmol/L: this level means small ketosis or mild ketosis. With these levels in blood, it is possible to generate energy through the process of burning fat. Nonetheless, if your goal is to lose weight, it is not yet at the appropriate level. Therefore, this level allows you to control the weight of the person.

3. The level of ketones in blood between 1.5 mmol/L and 3 mmol/L: By having this concentration of ketones in the blood we can consider that we are at the optimal level of ketosis in our body. Being this the level sought by people who make ketogenic diets. At this point, we can take advantage of the ketogenic level. Hence it is recommended to increase both physical and mental activities, in order to get the higher benefits of the keto. When this concentration of ketones is reached, our body will have a better condition to burn fat in an extremely efficient way, thus achieving weight loss.
4. The level of concentration of ketones in blood between 3 mmol/L and 8mmol/L: It is no longer good for the body since the objectives of the ketogenic diet are exceeded. At this
5. point, the results of it are not very positive because it does not have the same efficiency of using fat to generate energy. This level indicates that the body is not functioning properly. For example, the body is not sufficiently hydrated. For people who have a disease, such as type 1 diabetes, the problem may be linked to blood glucose and should be taken into account the level of insulin in their body.
6. The concentration of ketones in blood exceeds 8 mmol/L: This level is alarming since the level of concentration is extremely high for any human being. These values are not due to any ketogenic diet. These cases are found in patients with type 1 diabetes that are not controlled, being its main cause the low levels of insulin. In this case, it can be considered that the patient is in ketoacidosis due to a large amount of ketones in the blood, thus causing vomiting, nausea, and some other symptoms. This situation requires immediate medical treatment.

Already observing all the importance that ketones have in our bodies, we can say that they play a fundamental role in it. The ketones we are interested in are those generated by the liver after the decomposition of fat. But of course, this only happens at the time that the body does not have enough glucose to produce energy from it.

CHAPTER 3: WHAT HAPPENS TO YOUR BODY WHEN YOU GO KETO?

By applying the ketogenic diet as a lifestyle, our body goes into a metabolic state that is called ketosis in which our organism feeds entirely on fats.

Ketosis is nothing more than a state in which our body produces large amounts of substances, which function as a source of energy once carbohydrates are eliminated from our diet.

This could be seen as a state in which our organism guarantees its own survival without carbohydrates, learning to use fat as energy in the absence of the glucose substance. In this way our body, mainly our brain not only uses the fat stored in the blood but also feeds on the fats we eat in our food.

DIFFERENCES BETWEEN KETOSIS AND KETOACIDOSIS

It is very important not to confuse the state of ketosis with the state of ketoacidosis. The second one occurs when in our organism there are excesses of ketone molecules, and the body is unable to eliminate them through urine, making our organism enter a metabolic acidity that could be considered very severe and even fatal.

Ketoacidosis could be a very frequent risk that all those who suffer from diabetes disease could suffer, being fatal for their organism if it is not treated correctly.

BENEFITS OF KETOSIS

This condition allows our body to access fats found mainly in our bloodstream and the rest of the body. That is why it could be considered an effective way to lose weight.

Ketosis, in addition to allowing us to burn fat faster, gives us a feeling of satiety, reducing our appetite in a considerable way. In this sense, ketosis can help prevent cardiovascular disease.

- The brain: Containing high-fat substances, this provides certain curative properties for diseases such as epilepsy and even neurodegenerative diseases. Besides, has a great impact on the mood.
- In some cases, ketosis can influence diseases such as diabetes.
- Skin improvements related to the acne can be observed, as these ketone substances function as anti-inflammatory for the body.
- It can improve polycystic ovary syndrome and even fertility problems. By avoiding large intakes of insulin, the body increases androgen hormones (especially testosterone) thus increasing fertility.
- The ketogenic diet can improve glucose metabolism by lowering levels of sugar in our bloodstream and may even improve blood pressure and glycaemic profile.
- Ketonic molecules by activating our lipolytic metabolism effectively increases antioxidants in our body.
- Brain injuries: Studies reveal that this type of diet is capable of reducing some brain injuries that have been suffered as a result of an accident causing a more effective recovery in the patient. Many studies conclude that it can benefit Parkinson's and cancer patients, helping to treat some light types of these diseases and reducing the growth of cancerous tumors.

RISKS OF KETOSIS

Ketosis despite having its great advantages also has some side effects. That is why before starting a ketogenic diet (or any other type of diet) you should go to a specialist to examine your physical conditions and help you to develop a meal plan that can fit your needs. In this way, you will be preventing certain side effects such as:

- Sweating with a strong odor: This happens when ketone cells are eliminated.
- Bad Breath: By having excess of ketone molecules, these will be released through our breath. In the case of suffering this effect, it is recommended to consume a lot of water in order to reduce it.
- Headache: This can happen while our body adapts to our new food routine since our brain will need glycogen for its functioning. We could even feel dizziness.
- Urine with an intense odor: This happens once the ketone bodies are eliminated through the urine, which is why its odor and color can become strong.
- Lack of appetite: By decreasing carbohydrates and increasing protein and fat, our body changes the way it digests food. So we might notice that our appetite is decreasing as our body is getting used to this lifestyle.

- Arrhythmias: When so many changes take place in our organism, it is possible to show some cardiac problems.

Due to the changes that our organism suffers, it is very common that vomiting, decay, nausea, and even respiratory difficulty occur.

By reducing the consumption of fiber such as grains and cereals, we could present constipation.

Usually, this type of diet is not recommended for a period longer than three months because we could feel constantly tired and even lower our performance in everyday activities.

If we want to go back to the nutritional regime we used to have, it is important to follow the same steps we followed to start with the ketogenic diet. We must go back to carbohydrates gradually because a drastic change could cause problems such as sudden weight gain.

CHAPTER 4: HEAL YOUR BODY

Everybody knows that people who make this diet seeks to lose weight. But it is also used to control some diseases. For those reasons it is important this chapter, that will talk about health.

At first, we want to give a small concept of what health is. According to the world health organization, it is "A state of complete physical, mental and social well-being, and not merely the absence of illness or injury", therefore we can say that health does not mean the absence of any disease. Instead, it means having a certain quality of life that allows us to live in a comfortable way and without so many worries. It is also contemplated to be in a good mental and social state because there are people that you may know who are physically healthy but always feel bad or are depressed. That type of person cannot be considered completely healthy, and in the long run, this has implications on their physical health.

Moreover, a small example of the implications that mental health has with physical wellness is stress because it can affect our health without us realizing. There are occasions in which we get extremely strong headaches caused by anxiety or pain. Sometimes we get muscle tension thanks to restlessness. Chest pain could be for lack of motivation or much pressure; fatigue is due many times thanks to feeling overwhelmed. Changes in sexual desire has implications with anger. Stomach discomfort can be linked to depression. Even sleep problems can be linked to all the previous problems. In addition, it has been proven that diseases such as cancer are often developed by the moods that people have, and also that the happier or mentally healthy the patient is, the better his recovery from disease is. For this reason, it is important to have good mental health, because no matter what we achieve with the ketogenic diet if we are going to have problems with our mental health.

Now that the topic of integral health is over, we can now fully focus on the benefits that keto diet has on our health.

The first thing to do is to reduce the consumption of carbohydrates, sugars and harmful fats, which affects our body for different reasons. The first two foods mentioned, become glucose and if you make a very high consumption of them; they could lead to diabetes. This does not mean that you can not consume carbohydrates, because they are one of the main responsible for energizing our body. The organs, for some of their vital functions, use the glucose into which carbohydrates are converted and thus generate many processes extremely necessary for our body. One of these processes can be when an athlete lifts weights. The muscle will need to use glucose to be able to grow or to synthesize the exercise done; but if the muscles are not able to find glucose in our body, the muscle will decrease in size, in other words, reducing body mass.

Our organs do other processes that need glucose. Nevertheless, that component can be substituted in order to do these vital functions. It is substituted by the ketones produced by the liver. An organ that satisfies these characteristics is the brain since its vital functions can be performed with ketones instead of glucose. A better example could be the previous one; muscles need glucose in order to process the exercise done. This process cannot be done by any other cell other than glucose, but if we are under the keto regime, some organ will have to donate its glucose and feed on ketones. This can be done by the brain as it is able to use ketones to perform its tasks, managing to give energy to muscles to perform their synthesis processes and not to lose muscle mass.

As you can see, glucose consumption is reduced, which means a substantial improvement in the case of people who suffers diabetes since there are some cases in which the patient can stop consuming insulin. There are also cases in which cancer patients were benefited. It is because cancer cells eat mostly glucose cells. Therefore, when eating ketogenically, the production of glucose is reduced, hence the cancer cells are unable to feed themselves. There are also some studies that reveal that the consumption of food recommended by the ketogenic diet helps patients when it comes to receiving chemotherapy or radiotherapy. Although the results are not yet conclusive, it can be said that the results obtained with the ketogenic diet are hopeful.

It is important to mention that it helps reducing overweight. Ketogenic diet's goal is to process fat and use it as energy. Therefore, when burning fat, we can lose weight, then you can lower the rates of overweight, being this one of the most common diseases in the United States and around the world.

When it comes to the brain, the keto diet is also remarkable. Thanks to the keto diet, some of the brain's functions have a better performance. First of all, it protects the brain function. According to studies, it has been discovered that the ketogenic diet could regenerate the in some occasions brain damage. These results were obtained after having done experiments on animals. The first that was done was to feed very old animals with the ketogenic diet. After some time, it could be observed that those animals who fed normally had more difficulty to perform different activities than the ones that were on the keto diet. Then, we can say that the brain works better with the ketones produced by the liver than with the glucose generated by eating carbohydrates or sugars.

At first sight, this diet can be seen as one of the bunch, which has the purpose of considerably reducing people's weight. That idea cannot be further from reality since its health benefits are incalculable. To tell one of the many benefits of keto we will go back to its beginnings. It was used in patients who suffered from epilepsy diseases; epilepsy is an electrical overactivity in some areas of the brain. There were cases in which the children did not respond correctly to the pills that were responsible for controlling the attacks. The solution was the keto diet. Amazing results were obtained as more than 10% of the children to whom this diet was prescribed stopped seizures while more than 100% of the people who suffered from epilepsy and used keto diet could reduce their seizure frequency to about half.

That was not magic, it was because this diet had very important implications related to epilepsy. When the body enters into the state of ketosis, the behavior of some genes of the brain are altered; some of them are responsible for making the energetic metabolism of the brain, thus causing seizures. Another extremely important result is that an abysmal improvement in the energy of the neurons found in the hippocampus could be observed; increasing the density of mitochondria found within the hippocampus.

As if this were not enough, it could also improve the condition of other patients who suffer from Alzheimer's, which is a degenerative disease. This disease will gradually damage the connections that occur in the brain. It affects people in a very tough way since they will lose their memory to the point of not being able to perform their daily or basic activities. But using the ketogenic diet, some of these conditions could be improved.

We cannot say that this stops or reverts the condition, but we can say that there are hopeful results when using this diet in those cases. Experimentations on animals have been made and some kind of healing and improvement were observed on their brains. Even some damage was reverted. This happens because when you enter the ketogenic state, it is possible to reactivate certain neurons and repair part of the brain damage. Additionally, we can see that it also takes care of the brain protecting the dendrites and axons improving a vital process. Dendrites and axons are in charge of brain connections so that the human body can make synapses.

Therefore, we can be sure that the ketogenic diet is not only able to make people lose weight but also allows them to upgrade their living conditions. If the patient suffers any kind of diseases such as cancer or diabetes, we can recommend to try the keto diet, obviously, with the help of an expert.

CHAPTER 5:
IS KETO FOR YOU?

Before trying any diet we suggest to investigate thoroughly in order to understand the consequences that it could have on our body. It is essential to know its fundamentals, advantages, and disadvantages.

It is crucial in order to know if a diet is suitable for our system or not. Because diets works differently for each person.

It is well known that this diet is low in carbohydrates, moderate in protein and high in healthy fat. That distribution is what helps us to reach ketosis; causing the liver to take fatty acids and transform them into ketones to feed itself and use them as energy sources.

This diet is based on a calorie ratio between which 60-75% covers fat intake, 15-30% covers protein intake and 5-10% covers carbohydrate intake.

Among the foods that are allowed in the ketogenic diet, we can mention fats and oils such as almonds, avocado, peanuts, olive oil, fish, pecans, and linseed. It is advisable to eat these proteins that come from an ecological origin such as meats that have been fed on grass, chickens raised in a free environment, fish and seafood, fatty dairy products such as cream, cream cheese, and cured cheeses. Among the recommended carbohydrates are almond butter, mushroom seeds, chocolate (preferably without sugar), consumption of coconut and its derivatives.

The only left step is to take into account the following aspects that could give us a preliminary evaluation to know if the ketogenic diet is convenient for our organism:

1. The keto diet has no restrictions in terms of calorie consumption, so it could be said that we could have freedom with that consumption.
2. The keto diet gives the feeling of being satisfied with meals for longer. This is very good because we do not limit ourselves to reducing our food. Instead, we feed ourselves with what is necessary and we are satisfied with it.
3. The keto diet helps us to have more energy and, although it is known that diets high in carbohydrates generate some kind of energetic decline after eating and that diets low in calories only generate hunger and stress, this diet avoids that by adapting to the fats it eliminates through the reserves and providing us with enough energy to not depend on

proteins and carbohydrates. With this, we can have a high energy level during the day and we will not be constantly tired.

In few words, we can say that with the help of the keto diet we contribute to improve our physical quality of life and contribute to our health with long-term effects as long as it is done correctly. All this without worrying about the rebound effect, in which, we lose weight quickly and we gain it back in the same way.

We will achieve this as long as we are willing to radically change our habits. Of course, occasionally we will be able to enjoy a pizza, a hamburger and even cookies at some meal of the day (this must be done very carefully).

The ketogenic diet is not only to feed ourselves in a healthy way, we also must be constant to get a good result. Our body will take its necessary time to process the changes and enter the state of ketosis (may occur within the first 24 hours or up to a week) and be able to begin its process of burning fat and using ketones as energy source.

If you suffer from problems tolerating certain foods high in fat, sugar problems, renal history or any other inconvenience, the ketogenic diet may adapt to your needs, but it is advisable to go to the specialist before making any change in your feeding habits.

It is important to know that ketones do not work the same way as glucose in our body and that is why we need a higher consumption of fatty acids. Doing this, the lack of glucose will be substituted, hence, fulfilling the function of reducing weight, improving our body, eliminating carbohydrates and avoiding the accumulation of useless fat.

It is well known that excess of sugars and carbohydrates are the main cause of obesity, since when fat accumulates it stagnates in our body and can cause serious problems and even have a fatal result in the long term.

All types of diet have their risks and that is why we must be attentive and know if it will fit our body because, otherwise, we can have harmful results.

It is also known that in order to enjoy good health it is important to drink plenty of water and consume varied foods in a balanced way, mostly fruits and vegetables.

CHAPTER 6: BENEFITS OF KETOGENIC DIET FOR WOMEN

In both women and men, the endocrine system is formed by organs and tissues that produce hormones. These hormones are natural chemicals that, after produced, will be secreted into the bloodstream to be used by other organs. It is the general process that our endocrine system performs.

The hormones will then control those organs to which they are destined. However, there are some organic systems that contain their own systems to regulate them without needing hormones.

Now, as women (as this book is aimed for you) get older, there will be particular changes in these hormonal control systems. What is going to happen is that some organs or tissues become sensitive to the hormones that control them, in other cases, the number of hormones that the body can produce decreases with age. Sometimes, it may happen that the hormones decompose or metabolize more slowly.

Knowing roughly what happens with our endocrine system, we can deduce that when endocrine tissue ages, it can produce less amount of hormones than it was likely to, or perhaps it does produce the same amount of hormones but at a slower rate.

Among the hormones that can probably decrease over the years, is the Aldosterone hormone. This hormone is responsible for regulating the balance of liquids and electrolytes in the body. Other hormones are the growth hormone and renin hormone. In women, the levels of estrogen and prolactin generally decrease considerably over the years.

The ketogenic diet induces a metabolic condition that has been called "physiological ketosis" by Hans Krebs and has also been described as an adaptive mechanism preserved within all higher-order organisms to ensure survival during periods of starvation, illness or energy stress.

The ketogenic diet has been used with tremendous success in diseases such as epilepsy. In the case of women, most use it to lose weight and it is due to problems caused mainly by accumulated fat in the body. That accumulated fat has side effects that affect our health, so the main cause of the implementation of this diet nowadays is to lose weight.

When the processes of hyperinsulinism and hormonal alterations are occurring in women, they are not able to ovulate, considering that the entire menstrual cycle is disturbed. This is attributable to a hormonal imbalance between estrogens and progesterone; imbalance that leads to an increase in androgens which destabilizes the entire menstrual cycle and causes women not to ovulate. This increase in androgens starts to affect women's menstruation and other hormonal problems. With the keto diet, these imbalances disappear, actually, there are many gynecologists who recommend it. Surprising results have been seen in women after about ten months of following the keto diet and the evolution and improvement of the "polycystic ovary syndrome".

The entire female hormonal system improves as a result that female hormones are formed from a molecule called "cholesterol". Cholesterol is the basis for the formation of all steroid hormones like glucocorticoids, androgens, estrogens, and progesterone.

This diet is excellent for the liver and the menstrual cycle of women depends directly on hormones meaning that the keto diet helps you significantly for your entire hormonal system. As a consequence that the menstrual cycle is regulated, the ovulation improves, bleeding decreases and in fact, menstrual cramps improve significantly. In the case of women who are in menopause, the diet also helps, now that the production of female hormones is increased. Thus making this stage of the woman's life more bearable.

The keto diet improves brain health, headaches problems, and degenerative diseases. Neurologists are asking women to do the keto diet because, with the reduction of carbohydrates, migraine problems and headaches decrease and, in many cases, it eradicates the disease.

Women also notice changes in their skin such as improvements in acne by cause of reducing processed fats. Improvements have also been observed in skin color, in the decrease of blackheads, and even eye bags. That is why it is currently one of the most implemented diets in the world. All the studies that have been made, based on the diet, show satisfactory results. The life quality of each person who applies it is noticeable and that is why, when you start to apply this nutritional method, you do not want to stop it.

So to finish, we can say that, although it is quite difficult to start this diet and follow each one of the indications as it is really hard to eliminate carbohydrates and sugar from your daily foods, once your body is detoxified from all the anti-nutrients that you have consumed for many years, it will not want to return to consume these foods. When you start with these changes in your habits, your organism will enter into the state known as "keto-adaptation". After that, the changes in your body will start to occur gradually. Do not hesitate on going keto but first talk to a specialist.

CHAPTER 7: USING KETO DIET TO CONTROL OR PREVENT AGE-RELATED CONDITIONS

As the organism ages, it is exposed to different disorders. Those disorders can be both physical and mental depending on each person and their physiology. The changes that occur with age are particularly different according to each person.

At the age of 20, it is very likely to have or show diseases or disorders that could be due to congenital or degenerative diseases such as multiple sclerosis, eating disorders that lead, as explained above, to cardiovascular diseases, diabetes, and some others.

From the age of 40 onwards, people tend to suffer from heart diseases and cancer, being those the main cause of deaths. Statistics especially indicate that at these ages the majority of women presents breast and pelvic cancer, and regardless of the genre, skin cancer, cancer of the colon, rectum, and prostate.

From the age of 50, it is common to see cases of prostate cancer, as well as obesity, and vision problems. During their 60's, people begin to suffer from bone problems, osteoarthritis, osteoporosis, problems associated with cognitive impairment, Alzheimer's and even Parkinson's disease.

As people get old, if they do not have healthy habits, they are probably going to suffer from one of the diseases or disorders mentioned above. Sugar is an important element in these diseases, as it can alter the cellular environment of our body and thus the destruction or mutation of cells. For that reason, every day there are more and more advertisements that want to encourage citizens to opt for organic food and healthy eating, free of sugars, processed foods, and gluten.

It is difficult to think that after so many years of consuming sugar, now we have to eliminate it from our diet. But if we go back to the past we can remember that our ancestors had longer lives than the actual ones.

Visits and explorations have been made to distant towns in different countries where the entire population has life expectancies of more than a hundred years. When they were questioned about what kind of food they had, the answers were always the same. They fed with the fruits produced by nature, vegetables, tubers, meats, fish, and fruits free of pesticides, gluten, and long-lasting chemicals.

In this context, there are worldwide campaigns to raise awareness of humanity in favor of extending our lives.

The approach of the ketogenic diet goes towards those theories. The fact that we can feed ourselves with food produced by nature sounds incredible. Indeed, physiologically talking, our organism does not need carbohydrates to work, regenerate, nor to survive; neither does need alcohol nor sweets. However, they are the most consumed products these days.

The keto diet eliminates the consumption of processed sugar and this step is important. Positive changes have been observed, such as improvements in disorders coming from age, diabetes, hypertension, polycystic ovaries, Alzheimer's, Parkinson's, and other pathologies.

For this reason, although the most commonly consumed food by humans today are carbohydrates, we must lower their consumption. Their consumption produces glucose in our bloodstream and that energy is not always adequate to feed our body, as it has been observed that when the body feeds on ketones, it is better fed.

In this sense, to have a higher cellular longevity, you should feed ketogenically. This will make your body able to work with the energy produced by ketones. Up to this point, your organism will have burnt accumulated fat from our body

It should be noted that the metabolism changes at around 28 years of age. This is due to hormonal aging and progressive decrease in the production of growth hormone, and the increase in insulin.

Added to this, the food habits that are carried out at present and the lack of exercise accelerates the accumulation of fat and lowers muscle mass. This produces overweight, cellulite, flaccidity, deformities, and so on. As we can see, these hormones are fundamental in the changes produced by age, and the keto diet mainly seeks an increase in the HCG hormone and a decrease and control of insulin.

For example, one of the main problems in older adults is the loss of muscle mass. This happens as a result that the body is no longer able to generate enough glucose; for that reason, the muscles cannot use the same amount of glucose to perform the job of muscle maintenance or the increase in muscle mass when exercising. Then, gradually, due to the lack of glucose generation, the body of older people will lose muscle mass.

That is why making a diet low in carbohydrates and rich in fat, as the keto diet, will modify the way our body works. As there are processes within our body that are done exclusively with the glucose of our blood, others can be done with both ketones and glucose. Muscles use glucose exclusively, but the brain, which is the organ that consumes the most energy can use both. Therefore it consumes the most glucose in a normal food plan, but in the case of a ketogenic food plan, so many ketones are produced that it will feed on them. Because of this, the glucose stored in the bloodstream will be sent to the muscles so that they can maintain body mass.

But we have to be careful with this because we do not want to say that it is impossible to lose muscle mass since there are people who will have very positive results when maintaining muscle mass, but some will not. Saying that all people will react the same to the diet is false.

Something that happens a lot in older adults is the lack of energy. This is because, when reaching a certain age, the body does not work the same way. This can happen either because the body does not secrete the same amount of insulin anymore, so we can't burn all the glucose in our body, generating less energy; or our body does not process the food as it used, generating a lower amount of glucose in the blood that leads to a reduction of energy levels. The solution to those problems could be migrating to another meal plan, in this case, as you might expect, we recommend the ketogenic diet. To lower the consumption of carbohydrates and sugars, and to increase drastically the consumption of fats, will make you able to enter the state of ketosis, thus feeding us through the ketones that could act in a more efficient way in our body. That's why you can hear or see older adults who look very well physically since all this is thanks to food.

Statistically, there have been experiments related to longevity and the keto diet. Hopeful results were obtained, however, experiments have only been made on mice, but it has been shown that their life expectancy increases by thirteen percent due to their high-fat diet compared to those who are fed with carbohydrates. Nonetheless, the most interesting point is not only that they live longer, but they do it better since they do it free of illness and diseases.

Seeing all the benefits that can bring to older adults this type of food we can only recommend you to consume it, of course, always under the supervision of your trusted doctor It can help you to upgrade your energy and thus feel more vitalized. With this, you will have a better functioning of the brain, among other things extremely important for the proper functioning of our body.

CHAPTER 8: SUPPORTING BASIC BODY SYSTEMS

When we talk about ketosis, it's just a natural state that occurs when the body feeds mostly on fat when following a low-carbohydrate diet. Ketosis has benefits but also has its possible side effects.

Ketosis is the process where the body produces small energy molecules called ketones, which are known as energy for the body and are used when there is a reduced amount of sugar in blood (glucose). In the human body, specifically in the liver, ketones are produced from fats and then used as energy. The brain does not feed exclusively on glucose, therefore, we can really say that the brain burns carbohydrates when you consume them in the form of glucose, however, if you consume few carbohydrates, the brain will have no problem using ketones instead of carbohydrates. Ketosis is important because the brain consumes a large amount of energy daily, but does not feed directly from fats, it does from ketones.

This function is essential for basic survival, otherwise, as the body stores a supply of glucose product of carbohydrates from one or two days, the brain stops doing its functions after a couple of days without food. After a while, it would have to convert muscle proteins into glucose, but this process is very inefficient to maintain brain function; a situation that would cause the organs to atrophy quickly, due to the absence of food. Luckily, the human body has evolved to be more intelligent, it has fat deposits that can serve to survive several weeks, of course, this being a very extreme case. Anyways, it must be a trained person because not everyone can do it.

When the brain has the opportunity to feed on ketones made from our body fat, many people feel more energy and mental focus, which also accelerates fat burning and in turn, it tries to lose weight.

Ketosis has different benefits that it can provide to the body and the brain; one of the first benefits is to give an unlimited supply of energy, increasing mental and physical performance, and in turn, reducing hunger, facilitating weight loss without so much effort. In addition, in order for the body to enter into ketosis, it is necessary to consume few carbohydrates, effectively correcting type 2 diabetes. Ketosis has been used to control epilepsy and, even without medication, it shows great potential to treat other medical conditions such as acne, and even treat cancer.

For your body to enter into ketosis it is necessary low levels of glucose, since it is our main source of energy. That is going to force our body to look for another food, being it the stored fats in our body. To achieve this, it is essential to follow a strict diet low in carbohydrates as the ketogenic diet. To intensify the ketosis, you can effectively add intermittent fasting.

To recognize if the body is entering into ketosis, it is possible to measure it by a sample of urine, blood or breath. There are also other signs that will be seen without a test; we can say that one of the symptoms is dry mouth and increased thirst and urine.

Keto breath: this means that your body, through the breath, has a smell similar to the nail polish remover; that smell is also felt in the sweat when exercising, most of the time it is temporary. Other indicators but in a positive way, are reduced hunger and increased energy.

As has been said earlier, to achieve a state of ketosis it is necessary to restrict carbohydrates as they become glucose and the body proceeds to use it to energize the brain and other organs. But going fully into the relationship that has ketosis with the body and benefits from it, we can see the following:

- Keto diet and heart: As we all know, the keto diet is capable of making a very considerable loss of weight, resulting in burning fat in industrial quantities. That reduces cardiovascular risks as they often depend on whether the person is obese or also if he has very high blood pressure. As it lowers cholesterol also reduces the chances of having a better protection against heart diseases. Another extremely useful thing about keto diet is that autophagy is increased; it is a way of cellular cleaning, which is great to help our body. Finally, while it is true that it is required to eat few carbohydrates and many fats, it is not recommended to eat bacon every day, but with moderation. The fats that are recommended are the avocado, olive oil, and other sourced of good natural fats that are good for our body.
- Keto and the brain: In addition to the benefits we already know of the ketogenic diet and brain diseases, such as Alzheimer's or epilepsy, we can get other uses of it for the brain such as that it can increase memory capacity. It can be used in older adults or people of any age. It also helps to increase brain capacity because thanks to experiments that were conducted on fat or old animals, with the ketogenic diet they responded better than those who were not fed that way. On the other hand, the ketogenic diet has obtained positive results in people who suffer from congenital hyperinsulinism, which produces hypoglycemia; disease that could cause brain damage. At the time of using this type of feeding, many problems have disappeared in some persons. As if that wasn't enough, it has also been the solution for many patients who suffer from migraines, reducing very

often the events of migraine thanks to the low-carbohydrate diet. Patients with Parkinson's have been also benefited from the consumption of the keto diet. These results were seen thanks to some studies that were conducted on this type of patients who were submitted to these diets for at least four weeks. Of those patients, forty-seven percent have reported that they feel better, and the symptoms have decreased. Finally, patients who suffered some brain damage can also visualize an improvement thanks to the ketogenic diet. That improvement attributed to the fact that it is responsible for increasing the connections between the dendrite and axons, which generates better communication between neurons, trying to regenerate the affected area.

CHAPTER 9: DIABETES PREVENTION

Before talking about what might refer to keto in diabetes, it will be necessary to define some concepts.

WHAT IS DIABETES?

It is known that diabetes is a disease in which the level of sugar in blood, also known as glucose, increases disproportionately. This glucose is the main source of energy in our body and comes from the food we eat in our daily meals.

Insulin is the hormone produced by the pancreas to help drain that sugar in our blood and thus allow the cells to move in order to function as energy to our body.

In the case of diabetic patients, the body is not able to produce insulin and in this way the glucose remains accumulated in the blood, being unable to reach the cells, causing dangerous and even deadly results for the person.

Over time, the excess of glucose in the blood can cause eye damage, damage to the nervous system, and damage to the renal system. It can also cause heart diseases, stroke and patients can even be amputated from a part of their body for damage suffered (due to excess glucose).

TYPES OF DIABETES

Type 1 Diabetes

This type of diabetes is one in which the body does not produce insulin on its own because of the immune system attacks and destroys the cells that are produced by the pancreas. This disease can appear at any age, but it is mostly diagnosed in children and young adults who must take a certain amount of insulin each day in order to control the sugar levels.

When a person with type 1 diabetes has a low-carbohydrate and high-fat diet, they can stabilize their blood glucose levels. However, this must be monitored constantly as it can cause hypoglycemia.

Type 1 diabetes may be seen as an autoimmune disease (the body destroys itself by mistake). You are at risk for diabetes if you have a family history of type 1 diabetes. This type of diabetes can occur at any age, but it is much more common in childhood.

Type 2 diabetes

This type of diabetes is one in which the body does not produce adequate insulin to control glucose levels. Most type 2 diabetes occurs as a result of a person who has a disordered lifestyle when it comes to food. It can appear at any age, and there are even cases of people who have been diagnosed since childhood.

A person is at risk for type 2 diabetes if he or she has had pre-diabetes or has overweight and does not do any physical activity. This disease is usually diagnosed in people over 40 years of age and in some cases, it is diagnosed in people whose family tree has had this disease.

Gestational diabetes

This type of diabetes occurs in some women during pregnancy and even disappears after childbirth in some cases. However, if a woman has had gestational diabetes, she is much more likely to have type 2 diabetes at some point in her life (either in the short or long term).

A woman is at risk for gestational diabetes if she is overweighted, older than 25, or have a family history of type 2 diabetes. It can also influence if she has the hormonal disorder of polycystic ovary syndrome.

This type of diabetes usually goes away after childbirth, but the baby is more likely to have type 2 diabetes or obesity in his or her lifetime.

As we have been talking about, the ketogenic diet is one that is based on a diet of high fat consumption, moderate protein consumption, and very low carbohydrate consumption. When our body begins to consume glucose that is stored on it, it tries to find a way to get another source of energy, which in this case would be body fat.

This is why it is considered that the ketogenic diet in addition to helping to lose weight, can help regulate glucose levels by taking advantage of excess fat found in the body. Studies have shown that the ketogenic diet can influence up to 60% in the improvement of insulin in the body.

When a person who has diabetes (regardless type 1 or type 2) avoids carbohydrates in his or her dietary routine, which are the main factor in elevating blood sugar levels, he or she may be able to decrease medications to control these levels over time. This is because by not eating food that becomes glucose, the body will be able to respond by its own to insulin.

When starting this diet it is very important to keep track of glucose levels with a specialist, because if the person takes the same dose of insulin (that was medicated before starting the diet) when eating a low-carbohydrate diet, it could cause hypoglycemia which can be very harmful to health.

As we already know, it is not possible for two people suffering from diabetes to have the same dietary approach since they may share disease, but the body's way of reacting of each one is not the same. Ketogenic diets serve the purpose of improving the digestive system by eating healthy as long as it is followed correctly. This will be connected to the patient's physical condition.

There will always be some risks that need to be taken into account if you are under medical treatment. It is very important that under these conditions the patient is fully prepared to assume a diet so demanding that should not have any fault because its consequences can be serious; causing kidney problems, hypoglycemia, ketoacidosis, and kidney diseases. It could be even fatal.

IS THE KETO DIET SUITABLE FOR PEOPLE WITH DIABETES?

Some studies have shown that the keto diet is able to improve the health of some people suffering from this disease and even, in some cases, the minority has been able to improve insulin sensitivity.

Many people see this type of diet as a therapy for the treatment or improvement of the disease; however, this result only applies to some people. Due to the different body types, different patients do not always get the same results.

A person who is not willing to follow such a specialized and strict diet is not going to be able to obtain as goods results as a person who followed this type of diet properly.

What do we mean by that?

Once explained all the factors that influence, you could conclude that the keto diet is highly recommended by experts and people who suffer from diabetes, as they have achieved very positive results in their body and other personal aspects. However, it is very delicate to follow this type of diet, because if you do not have the necessary disposition it could be very dangerous. A slight mistake can damage your health and make a lot of damage.

CAN THE KETO DIET PREVENT DIABETES?

Some studies indicate that the keto diet might, in some way, influence the prevention of this disease (at least as far as type 2 diabetes is concerned) for the person whose purpose is to lead a healthy life. However, many times, this disease is diagnosed from childhood and any type of factor can influence (some failure in the body or possible family inheritance).

Diabetes can be prevented and (if you have it) also controlled up to a point where you will not depend entirely on medications. Of course, this will always depend on the person with the disease and their willingness to change their eating habits.

It is relevant that we are aware that when we make a type of diet in which less than 50 grams of carbohydrates are consumed per day, our body enters the state of ketosis to obtain energy through the burning of fat.

It is crucial for people with type 1 diabetes to be able to differentiate between ketosis and ketoacidosis as the last one can be dangerous because of the lack of insulin. It is also recommended to start with a low-carbohydrate diet in a less strict way (at least 50 grams per day initially) and adapt it to your taste over time.

While people with type 2 diabetes can greatly improve their health condition to such an extent that they can completely overcome the insulin injection, a person with type 1 diabetes will still need to continue injecting their insulin but maybe in a smaller amount.

CHAPTER 10: DIETARY EXCHANGE THROUGH THE MENSTRUAL CYCLE

All women possess hormones, which are regulated by three main glands; hypothalamus (located in the center of the brain), pituitary (located in the brain), and adrenal glands (located at the top of the kidneys). These glands are responsible for the rest of the hormones to be in proper balance, thus generating an HPA (hypothalamus pituitary adrenal axis) which is responsible for controlling stress levels, moods, emotions, digestion, the immune system, sexual desire, metabolism, and even our energy levels.

Calorie intake, stress, and physical exercise can cause these hormonal glands to become very sensitive, so it should be considered that a low-carbohydrate diet could affect the body significantly, these changes would be reflected in the attitude.

It is known that long-term stress is capable of generating very serious damage to the body, as the overproduction of cortisol and norepinephrine creates an imbalance in the body that increases the pressure on the hypothalamus and adrenal glands. This pressure causes a dysfunction of the HPA axis.

Referring to adrenal fatigue the most common symptoms that could be seen are fatigue, weakness in the immune system and a very high risk of presenting health problems.

The adrenal fatigue, being a little similar to the suprarenal fatigue has a series of symptoms, between which we can emphasize: fatigue, depressed or weak immune system, possibility of suffering hypothyroidism, inflammation, diabetes, and mood disorders in the long term; being these very serious for the health.

Many times the increase in cortisol levels is thanks to the fact that the person is submitted to a low-carbohydrate diet. As we already know, this is very different in comparison to a moderate-fat diet and for this reason, this type of diet can cause a much greater alteration of stress levels in women than in men.

By consuming few carbohydrates, in addition to generating a noticeable alteration in stress levels, could produce other discomforts such as irregular menstrual cycles or amenorrhea (this means the absence of menstrual cycle for 3 months or more). Amenorrhea is presented by the low levels of many different hormones such as the release of gonadotropin (GNRH) which is responsible for initiating the menstrual cycle and if this failed, would generate a collapse in all (or most) sex hormones, fsh, lh, estrogen, progesterone, and testosterone.

Another possible cause of amenorrhea is the low levels of leptin (a hormone produced by fat cells). According to experts, it is mentioned that in women, a certain level of leptin is very necessary to maintain a normal function in the menstrual cycle in order to maintain the regular functioning of reproductive hormones.

Low calorie or carbohydrate intake may cause leptin levels to be completely eliminated, resulting in an irregular menstrual cycle. It is very common for underweight women to be the most vulnerable to low levels of these hormones. Amenorrhea usually appears after a time on a low-carbohydrate diet.

When the keto diet is made, different corporal changes are experienced; but not all of them are always negative. The keto diet could be very useful for those women who suffer from POS (polycystic ovary syndrome), this disorder is the one that suppresses the development of ovaries and the liberation of the ovules.

Many of the experimental data indicate that those patients with POS who start the keto diet, manage to recover a regular menstrual cycle and can also contribute to fertility.

When suffering from POS, the excess of insulin in a woman's body is capable of causing a considerable increase in her androgen and testosterone levels, which generates a limitation in the production of estrogens and the body's capacity to ovulate.

When a woman is on the keto diet, she must prepare herself (both physically and psychologically) for the changes she is going to go through.

As mentioned above, it is quite possible that among the changes that may occur is the devastation in the menstrual cycle due to sudden weight loss (caused by alteration of the balance of estrogen and progesterone).

However, an irregular period could not be a worrying change since the menstrual cycle could stop completely; this happens a lot in women who lose a lot of weight and are very thin because their body is more vulnerable to amenorrhea (absence of menstrual cycle) due to anovulation (lack of ovulation).

It is important to note that these problems are very likely to be attributed to sudden weight loss in response to the keto diet. Otherwise, it is very likely due to other factors such as very low body mass index, a low-calorie diet and could even be presented by excess exercise; causing the decrease of some hormones that regulate ovulation, bringing consequences of irregularity.

The lack of carbohydrates could be another key factor in ovulation problems as it directly affects the luteinizing hormone which is released by the brain to help regulate ovulation. When this hormone is directly affected, hypomenorrhea (short, light menstrual cycles) may occur.

Surely you must be wondering... How many carbohydrates must a woman ingest to avoid these types of problems?

It is not really possible to indicate an exact amount since each body assimilates food intake in different ways.

In its majority, the nutritionists indicate to consume between 15 and 30% of carbohydrates, this would be the equivalent to between 75 and 140 grams daily of calories in the form of carbohydrates; nevertheless, there are cases of women in which a diet low in carbohydrates tends to benefit their organism much more (those that suffer from POS).

But, there are cases of women who are recommended to consume between 100 and 150 grams of carbohydrates a day, these can be all those:

- Mothers who are breastfeeding.
- Women who have suffered an interruption of their menstrual cycle.
- Women who wish to gain weight.
- Women who have practiced the Keto diet for a very long time.
- Pregnant women

This type of food intake will be recommended to all those women who suffer from the cases mentioned above; besides, this routine will achieve a harmony in their mood and provide a good amount of energy to perform in their daily activities.

From here, we could conclude that the keto diet can be very useful for those women who suffer from polycystic ovary syndrome which, as mentioned above, is a hormonal disorder that prevents the ovaries from releasing ovules (thus allowing a regular menstruation).

We also know that in some cases women who have made the keto diet, have managed to get a regular period, as well as helping the fertility of women.

Why is this?

This is because, with polycystic ovary syndrome, excess of insulin in the female body increases the levels of androgens and testosterone limiting the production of estrogen and also the ability to ovulate.

In conclusion, the keto diet besides promoting weight loss also helps the symptoms of polycystic ovary syndrome. It is very important to see a specialist before undergoing this diet because, as you could see it can cause a lot of hormonal changes and it is necessary to be prepared for it.

It is also highly recommended not to focus solely on the keto diet but to complement it with another style (as recommended by your specialist). So, in addition to maintaining an ideal weight, it helps you to follow this in the long term and get benefits for your body since the key to a regular menstrual cycle is to follow a diet that adapts to your needs

CHAPTER 11: KETOGENIC DIET AND FERTILITY

One of the greatest illusions that women have is giving birth to a child. The great majority of women dream about it; they wish to raise him until they are grown up and want to feel proud of them. Unfortunately, not all women are capable of doing that for different reasons, as we will see below, they can be the following:

- Having untreated sexual diseases.
- Having blocked Fallopian tubes. This does not allow sperm to reach the ovule, thus not allowing the stage of gestation.
- Lack of ovulation. If the woman does not generate ovules, then it is not possible to make the union sperm-ovule, which have to unite to generate life.
- Poor quality ovules. This means that they are not able to generate a baby, no matter how many unions are made with the sperm.
- The way in which the uterus is found limits or makes it difficult to have a fertilized ovule.
- Uterine fibroids. Represents having some type of tumors, which are not cancerous, which are like walls or muscle cells, located in the walls of the uterus, they do not allow sperm to reach the ovule.
- Having an endometriosis. Meaning that you get the same tissue that covers the interior of the uterus outside it. We say this, because all the tissue that covers the inside of the uterus, also grows outside it; hence growing in places where it should not; leading to fertility problems.
- Having polycystic ovaries. This indicates that the woman has a disease, which has extremely high levels of hormones specifically androgens. This situation not only affects fertility but also affects the effect of having menstrual irregularities, acne problems and an increase in body hair.

While it is true that the ketogenic diet is not magical and it will not be able to heal all of the conditions it is true that it can help us with one of them; w with the polycystic ovaries. It is important to know perfectly the reason why it helps us and what it is about; since the explanation previously made is very ambiguous or simple. Therefore, it is better to explain it in a better way, so that we are able to talk about it properly.

The first thing is that this is a very common condition in women since it is based on a hormonal disorder in women who are at reproductive age. To start, women who have this condition have extremely irregular menstrual cycles, which can happen rarely or infrequently, or also present a period of menstruation quite long. In addition, generates an excessive level of hormone that is characteristic of men, which is called androgen. Thanks to all these conditions that can be suffered by having polycystic ovaries, small accumulations of liquid start to form. These accumulations can be blood, called follicles in the ovaries that may cause the ovules not to be generated in a normal or regular. Consequently causing fertility problems in women.

The first and very essential thing is to know if you have polycystic ovaries. This is done by observing yourself and verifying if you have a cumulus of symptoms; if you have them, it is recommended to go to a specialist doctor. Fortunately, this condition has treatment which means a great relief for women who have infertility because of the polycystic ovaries.

The first thing we can say is that these symptoms can be seen from the first menstruation happened in the woman. This occurs most of the time, but there is also the possibility that it occurs in an adult stage; nonetheless, the latter may be due to a significant weight gain. But it is important to emphasize that for you to have a real possibility of having polycystic ovarian syndrome, you must show at least two of these symptoms:

- A lot of androgen in your body. This can be seen in different ways, when we talk about the physical form, you can see to have an excess of facial hair or even body hair, but you can also see to have a lack of hair, being it a male pattern.
- Having polycystic ovaries. Which means that your ovaries are dilated, and also could have follicles around your ovules, thus causing a malfunction of the ovaries of women in an age of fertility.
- To have irregular menstrual periods. With this, we mean to present an extra menstruation that is not planned at all with the count of the twenty-eight days in order for the next menstruation to occur. It could also be a very big irregularity in the frequency that each one of your menstruations occurs; being these periods very short or very long. This can be the most common sign for the women who have the syndrome of the polycystic ovaries, this irregularity, could be that a woman has 16 or 7 menstrual periods in a year.

But the syndrome of polycystic ovaries does not appear suddenly, instead, it has some causes, this syndrome has factors which can contribute to deteriorate the situation of the ovaries as follows:

Having excess insulin in the blood: This happens, as you should know because our body is capable of processing the glucose in our body which is the main source of energy if we have a traditional diet high in carbohydrates and the hormone responsible for doing this is insulin; but as long as it is at normal levels in our body. But if this hormone is at a high level, causing the cells to be resistant to insulin, there will be a high level of sugar in the blood, which could cause an increase in androgens in our body thus producing a greater difficulty in ovulation.

Simply excess of androgen, and as we said previously, this causes a very large complication to be able to ovulate, so it becomes almost impossible to have a good fertility.

These causes can also be simply hereditary, therefore, the syndrome of polycystic ovaries can be simply because the woman has inherited this condition from her ancestors.

Little inflammation: this is measured by the production of white blood cells that generates our body, so we can combat an infection. Women who have such a condition have a type of little inflammation that will stimulate the polycystic ovaries which in the long run generate more androgens. Then, in addition to generating hormonal problems, can also generate problems generated with the heart and blood vessels.

When we see the statistics, and we observe the main causes of infertility in women, we can say that eighty percent of them have obesity, but also have insulin resistance and, as we know, having such conditions increases the amounts of androgens in our body. Being insulin resistance the major cause of polycystic ovarian syndrome. In fact, the latest statistics tell us that more than ninety percent of people who have hyperinsulinism, of course in women, have the syndrome of polycystic ovaries, being this a major problem when it comes to the fertilization process.

For this reason, we see that one of the main causes of polycystic ovarian syndrome is having high insulin, the product of having a high level of glucose in the blood and these levels of glucose in our blood are a product of a diet rich in carbohydrates or traditional food. Therefore, by making a considerable decrease in carbohydrates and sugars, we will lose a considerable amount of weight, but it decreases in a more than considerable way the level of glucose in our blood, thus decreasing one of the main causes of the syndrome of polycystic ovaries.

The first thing is that, at the time of losing weight by means of the ketogenic diet, it is possible to reduce in an extremely important way the inflammation. If you were focused enough during this chapter, you could have seen that the inflammation has a direct implication with the process of fertilization because if the woman is inflamed it is possible to get damage in the fallopian tubes, thus causing problems when fertilizing. For this reason, when making the keto diet, we can significantly lower the inflammation within our body, since this type of feeding recommends the consumption of foods that are anti-inflammatory and extremely healthy, thus achieving to lower the inflammation in our organism in such a way that we could unblock, the tube of the fallopian tubes. This will result in achieving an improvement in the possibility of getting pregnant; however, in case of having inflamed fallopian tubes, it is difficult to determine since it does not cause pain, only infertility. Therefore, a way to try to combat this condition is applying this type of diet.

On the other hand, the consumption of a ketogenic diet also allows to have better control of the hormones since the women who possess the syndrome of politic ovaries have a hormonal disorder. This disorder produces a high number of hormones that should be generated by the male gender, causing these problems in the ambit of the ovulation of the woman; for that reason, it is necessary to look for some alternatives to be able to control these hormones.

In this case, the keto diet does not stay behind and allows an exaggerated reduction in the amount of glucose in the blood which makes it possible to control insulin levels. As the person is doing a low consumption of carbohydrates, these glucose cells are not generated, thus achieving the regularization of hormones within the body of females. Moreover, there are specialists in the field that say that a decrease in weight, between five or ten percent, can involve better ovulation. With this, we can say that the ketogenic diet can help regulate hormonal behavior, leading to achieve something so wonderful like healing some women who suffered from infertility problems before doing the ketogenic treatment. There was an experiment that was made with four women, who had the illusion of being able to conceive a child but no matter how hard they tried or how many attempts they made, they had not been able. Surprisingly, after a few months of having started to eat a diet low in carbohydrates, but rich in fat, not only did they lose considerably their weight, but they also managed to rebalance their hormones, helping them to solve some of their infertility problems.

In this case, we can say that these infertility problems can be solved through the ketogenic diet, but by this, we do not mean that it can solve them all, only a few related to the syndrome of polycystic ovaries and overweight. As we have been saying through all the previous chapters, it is never too much to go to the doctor or a specialist to be able to make a treatment in which the woman is able to ovulate or to get to fertilize in order to reach the miracle of life.

CHAPTER 12:
BASIC RECIPES

As we know, the keto diet is a low-carbohydrate, high-fat diet plan. Applying this plan will make it possible to reduce weight and improve certain conditions considerably as we discussed before, like blood sugar levels and insulin levels and thus produce a transition in the body's metabolism where carbohydrates will be replaced by fat and ketones.

Now, which are the foods that we must avoid in order to successfully begin this plan?

- Cereals: corn, rice, wheat, barley, oats, grains, sprouts, amaranth, rye, among others.
- Legumes: common bean, chickpea, black bean, green pea lentil, broad bean.
- Starch: potato, carrot, yucca, sweet potato.
- Furtas: banana, papaya, apple, pineapple, orange, grape, mango, tangerine, fruit juices, nuts, fruit syrup, concentrates.
- Alcohol: beer, some wines, cocktails.
- Sugars: honey, agave nectar, maple honey, sugar, corn syrup, fructose, sugar cane.
- The foods that we should consume and that are also recommended in this diet are the following:
- Vegetables: broccoli, cauliflower, spinach, champignons, asparagus, eggplant, zucchini, brussels sprouts, lettuce, paprika, onion, tomato.
- Fats: butter or ghee, lard, homemade mayonnaise, coconut oil, olive oil, cream, dark chocolate, fatty cheeses that melt easily, avocado, nuts and seeds such as flaxseed and chia, almonds, coconut flour, coconut milk, and almond milk.
- Fruits: berries, blackberries, strawberries, blueberries, raspberries.
- Proteins: tuna, ham, chicken, turkey, eggs, sausage, salami, beef, pork, veal, bacon, fish preferably oily fish, duck, and seafood.
- Canned food can be consumed but you will first have to carefully read the ingredients and verify that they do not contain sugars, corn syrup or starch.

Once we have knowledge of the foods we should not eat and those that we should consume we can proceed to know some of the basic keto recipes. In this order of ideas, we are going to proceed to show some short but delicious simple recipes that we can prepare to begin to change our life plan and our diet.

KETO TORTILLAS WITH LINSEED

Ingredients:

- 300 grams of mozzarella cheese.
- 50 grams of ground linseed, if you have it in seeds you can blend it easily.
- 1 egg.
- Salt to taste.

Steps to follow:

First, we are going to melt the mozzarella cheese (we can do this in the microwave or in a satin). Once the cheese is melted, we are going to add the ground linseed and mix the two ingredients. Finally, we are going to add the egg and the salt. It is necessary to emphasize that everything must be mixed very well so that the tortillas are not left with undesired consistences.

Then, divide the mixture into several portions, depending on the amount that comes out and the number of people, and in a pan over medium heat extend the portions for about five minutes; when cooked, they must be turned with a spatula so that they can cook on the other side.

KETO TORTILLA WITH ALMOND FLOUR AND COCONUT

Ingredients:

- ¾ Cup of almond flour.
- 4 spoonfuls of coconut flour.
- 1 egg.
- Salt to taste.
- 2 spoonfuls of warm water.

Steps to follow:

Place all the ingredients in a bowl, mix and knead until you get a homogeneous dough that is wet to the touch because we do not want it to be liquid to be able to manipulate it.

If we see that the dough is too dry, we can add a little water and knead again and this way you will work with the consistence you want to.

Once you have the dough with the desired consistency, wrap it in a food plastic and let it rest for about 10 minutes.

Once it has rested enough time, we proceed to divide the dough in about eight portions or in the quantity that is wanted, according to the size of the tortillas that are wanted to make.

The tortillas can be given the round shape either with palms with the hands in a natural way or can be made with the tortilla machine or with a bakery roller, if available.

If we make it with the method of the palms, we are going to place the balls of dough in a waxed paper and it will be given the round form with the palms of the hand.

With the machine for tortillas, you will place the ball of dough in the middle with the waxed paper so that it does not stick and crush until you get the tortilla.

Another way is to place the dough balls in the middle of two sheets of wax paper and stretch them with the roller until they acquire the shape, size, and thickness we want.

If we want them to be totally round we can make use of the cutters that are used in pastry.

Later we will proceed to place them in the frying pan (preferably anti-adherent) to medium heat, and let cook for 30 seconds approximately or when we observe that it begins to cook and change color. Then, we turn them to cook on the other side for a few more seconds and so on until you finish the desired amount of tortillas.

EMPANADAS OF KETO MEAT

Ingredients:

For the dough:

- 1 ½ cup almond flour.
- 1 ½ Cup of mozzarella cheese.
- 100 grams of cream cheese.
- 1 egg.

For the Stuffing:

- 1 tablespoon of butter preferably Ghee or clarified.
- ½ Kg of ground beef, you can perfectly mix it with a little pork meat and it will give it a surprising taste.
- 1 tablespoon finely chopped onion.
- ½ chopped tomato.

- Salt to taste.
- Ground pepper to taste.
- Concentrated consommé of beef broth, this is optional to add some more flavor.

Steps to follow:

1. In a frying pan over medium heat add the butter, you can add a little chili if desired, onion, tomato, and let's fry for a few minutes over medium heat until you see that your ingredients are integrating and cooking.
2. Then add the meat, mix, season with salt and pepper to taste, and if we have beef broth, we add it and let all the ingredients cook and mix for about five minutes approximately or until you see that the ingredients are well mixed and cooked.
3. We are going to let the meat cook a little and dry, but not much so that it is a little juicy, then we are going to let it rest to use it to fill the dough and make empanadas.

For the dough:

1. Mix the cream cheese and mozzarella cheese in a bowl, we can melt the cheeses in the microwave or manually in a pot, the important thing is to melt them so they can mix well. After we have mixed the cheeses, we add the egg, mix well to add almond flour gradually, and we are going to mix until a manageable dough is obtained, then let it rest for a few minutes.
2. To make the empanadas we make a few balls, the size will depend on the size we want our empanada. Again, we can make tortillas with the palm of the hands, with the machine to make the tortillas or in its defect with the roller, as explained in the previous recipe.
3. Once the tortilla has been made, add the meat filling that we left to rest earlier. Fold the tortilla in half and seal the dough with the fork so that the filling does not come out.
4. Then place the empanadas in a tray with waxed paper and take it to the oven at 180 Celsius degrees for 15 minutes or until they are golden. And they are ready to taste.

KETO PIZZA

Ingredients:

- 200 grams of almond flour.
- 700 grams of grated mozzarella cheese.
- 75 grams of cream cheese.
- 2 eggs.
- 150 grams of salami.

- 150 grams of Pepperoni.
- 150 grams of ground beef.
- 50 grams of Ghee butter.
- 50 ml of unsweetened tomato paste.
- Salt to taste.
- Ground Oregano to taste.
- Garlic powder to taste.

Steps to follow:

1. The first thing we are going to do is preheat the oven to 200 Celsius degrees while we prepare the dough and pizza.
2. For the dough, we are going to melt the cream cheese and half of the mozzarella cheese, we can melt it as it is already known in the microwave or in a pot avoiding of course that the cheese burns. It only has to reach the necessary temperature so that it melts and the two cheeses can be mixed.
3. Once the cheeses are mixed we add the salt to taste, the almond flour, the eggs and we mix everything very well, only in case it is necessary to be able to achieve a better mixture we can place again our container in the microwave to melt the cheeses and to mix well.
4. In a pizza mold, place a waxed paper to prevent our dough to stick; we are going to extend the dough in the pizza mold. A way to extend perfectly the dough is with this technique: we are going to place the dough in the waxed paper and on top, we are going to place another sheet of waxed paper and stretch. Once reached the desired size remove the waxed paper from above and take the mixture to the oven for about 10 to 15 minutes at a temperature of 200 ºC until we see that it begins to roast a little.
5. For the filling of our pizza, we are going to stir fry the meat with the butter or if we prefer we can do it with olive oil.
6. Once the base of the pizza is golden brown, remove it from the oven and let it rest so that the cheese solidifies, then add the tomato paste mixed with garlic powder and oregano, add the ground beef, pepperoni, sliced salami, and finally the rest of the mozzarella cheese.
7. We put it back into the oven; this time for a few minutes because all we want is to melt the mozzarella cheese, let cool a little and it will be ready to eat. If we want, we can also add olives and mushrooms.

Ingredients:

- 1 clove of garlic.
- ½ Medium onion.
- 250 grams of natural preference sliced mushrooms.
- 1 tablespoon Ghee butter.
- 300 ml of whipping cream.
- 1 cup spinach.
- 1 pinch of salt to taste.

Steps to follow:

1. In a frying pan over medium heat add the butter and cook the finely chopped onion and garlic. When the onion has a transparent color, add the sliced mushrooms and stir constantly so that they do not stick until they are golden and caramelized.
2. Then we will add the whipping cream, the pinch of salt, and move carefully to incorporate until it boils.
3. When the boil breaks, add the spinach, stir and let cook for about two minutes so that the spinach is not overcooked.
4. All we have to do now if we want to; is to blend all the ingredients to obtain the cream. There are people who do not blend it and the flavor is just as wonderful, once the cream is obtained we serve it hot and enjoy.
5. If we get leftover cream, we can refrigerate it in a container with lid and save until the next time we want to consume, at that time, it can be heated in a frying pan over low heat. This recipe can also be used as a sauce to complement a chicken or pork and is equally delicious.

As we can see, it is easy to take this food plan and once we try the recipes we will realize that they are as tasty as the usual diets. It is crucial to try that the food is accompanied by nutrients that our body can absorb, such as spinach and vegetables, coconut oil and other foods that provide a good amount of vitamins and nutrients necessary for our body.

CHAPTER 13:
FOOD CHOICE

It is already known to us that if we eat the right diet we can reach the desired levels of ketosis and enjoy the many benefits that this provides.

That is why it is important to evaluate very well which foods we are going to buy when starting the ketogenic diet. The important thing is to choose products that, in addition to being allowed in the keto diet, provide us with the vitamins and minerals that our body needs because, as the cellular environment is regenerated and cleaned, we will have the ability to absorb all the nutrients from the food ingested.

Based on this, we are going to talk about some foods that are supposed to be consumed in this diet for the nutritional contribution they have for our body.

Whitefish, such as hake or similar fish are a good choice as they are lean options and very reduced in calories but with a high-quality protein for our body, especially for its high proportion of omega 3, essential for health.

The avocado is one of the few oily fruits sources of vegetable protein admitted by the keto diet and also widely used in this food plan for its big versatility when preparing a dish as it is used for salads, sauces, and even desserts. The avocado is a fruit considered an excellent antioxidant and rich in vitamins and minerals, with a natural fat that is widely used in these keto diets.

Vegetables are also allowed and widely recommended in the ketogenic diet; especially green vegetables. These green vegetables are source of vitamins and recommended fibers; in the specific case of spinach we have that it is a vegetable used in most keto dishes and it is because spinach, apart from containing fiber, has vitamin A, B1, B2, C, K, calcium, phosphorus, iron, folic acid, is rich in magnesium, zinc, and beta-carotene, the latter slowing the action of free radicals, making spinach to be considered as a natural anticarcinogen. Spinach can improve the functioning of the immune system and vision. As we already know, vegetables form most of the distribution of food that must be present in the daily dishes so it is necessary to ingest products of good quality and with a great contribution such as spinach.

In the case of vegetables, not all vegetables are allowed in the keto diet, this is because some of them have a high content of starch and carbohydrates that are processed by the body as sugar and, as far as we know, we must avoid it in this diet plan. That is the case of the potatoes, sweet potatoes and cassava, for example. However, there are other vegetables that are allowed since they are low in carbohydrates, such as cauliflower, broccoli, bell pepper, celery, cucumber, eggplant, and asparagus. Cauliflower is a highly recommended and used vegetable, low in carbohydrate and high in fiber and vitamin C.

When talking about cheeses, the first thing we are going to recommend is to consume organic and defatted cheeses coming from animals preferably fed with grass. It is important to be able to evaluate the nutritional information of the cheeses that are ingested, the lesser ingredients they have the better they are since there are many products that can have stabilizers that add carbohydrates and sugars to the cheeses.

A topic of discussion is the consumption of milk as it contains large amounts of carbohydrate so the milk allowed is from nuts; such as almond milk, and coconut milk without sugar. The detail is that many specialists do not recommend consuming those milks because to generate a glass of almond milk, it requires large amounts of almonds, thus exceeding the amount of fat you can ingest daily. You consume large amounts, of course, that is what it is recommended in the keto diet, but moderately. The same applies to almond and coconut flours.

In the case of clarified butter or Ghee, just like the oils allowed, its content is clearly fat without carbohydrates or proteins. In fact, more than 60% of the ketogenic diet is fat, so they are one of those that can be used with more confidence for the preparation of most dishes. It is recommended, as we have been saying previously, to choose good quality products and, currently, on the market there is a wide variety of them.

Nutritional yeast is a good ally of people who apply the ketogenic diet because when it is sprinkled on meals you get a delicious cheese flavor, it is also rich in vitamin B12 and is often used to make cakes and breads.

Another component of food that we can not leave behind and that we want to recommend is collagen. This can be found in the gelatine extracted from the broth of beef legs, for example. Collagen is the most abundant protein in mammals including humans. It is one of the most important components, especially in these processes in which people are losing weight and reducing sizes and is required to improve the elasticity of the skin. Collagen helps the skin, bones and connective tissues and represents almost a third of our total mass of protein.

That is why we strongly recommend consuming gelatine that is collagen in a natural way. The most commonly used is the gelatine made with beef legs broth, which contains a large amount of collagen protein.

There is an oil used in the ketogenic diet that has many properties and it is the MCT oil, it consists of concentrated caprylic acid and which is 8 times more concentrated than coconut oil.

MCTs are easy to absorb fatty acids that metabolize very quickly and are effectively converted into long-lasting energy for the brain and body, and help to increase energy, endurance, and mental concentration while in a low-carbohydrate or ketogenic state.

MCT oil increases metabolism and improves your body's ability to burn body fat as a fuel source. As MCT oil is naturally tasteless and odorless it can be easily mixed with food without altering its flavors. For those who are starting to consume this type of oil, it is advisable to start with half a teaspoon that can be added to the morning coffee or in the coffee with which you are going to break the fast for example.

The Himalayan Pink Salt is another good recommendation that you can add to the amount of products that you must acquire if you are going to start this diet since it is a salt that preserves all the essential minerals and electrolytes, promotes healthy pH levels in the body, contains natural iodine, improves circulation, and does not increase blood pressure. Otherwise, common salt is not recommended because its minerals are lost in the process of industrialization and it can cause high pressure in the body when consumed in excess; iodine in this type of salt is artificially added in and it also includes anti-glomerate compounds. So when consuming salt in our meals choose pink salt or Himalayan salt.

With all that we have been able to appreciate so far, we have that within the great variety of foods allowed, if we evaluate and investigate their enormous properties and, in addition, we look for different combinations of dishes or menus that we can do with them, we will not find ourselves in the need to get bored of this lifestyle. We have to learn why some vegetables, for example, are not allowed in the food plan, only in this way and acquiring the knowledge about nutritional content of each of the foods we consume, we acquire awareness and responsibility of not consuming it.

Let's talk about cereals. They have a certain quantity of starch, some have more than others, that are metabolized in our body in the form of sugar; something that we should not consume in the keto diet. So, this type of food should be avoided, such as the case of rice, and we can replace it with keto rice using cauliflower. There is a wide variety of options that we can do and try to adjust the plan, not only to our economic needs but also to the needs and requirements of our body.

In the case of alcohol, it is not recommended to consume beer, cocktails and some wines. In the ketogenic diet, some types of wines may be allowed, such as dry wine containing less than 0.5 grams of sugar per glass. Most wines are presentations of beverages with carbohydrate concentrations due to various fermentation processes such as glycerol, which has a minimal effect on blood sugar concentration or insulin levels. With this information, we can use the analogy that every time we consume a glass of wine we are drinking 2 grams of carbohydrates.

When applying the keto diet, if we want to achieve the benefits and be able to obtain the levels of ketosis; we must not only be aware that we must follow the indications of the ketogenic diet, but also have some examples and some knowledge that we must take into account when choosing foods. Knowledge like: which vegetables are not allowed and which are the consequences of their consumption. We must also evaluate which foods we will consume and why, what benefits it would be contributing to my diet. If we do this process in a planned way organizing a weekly menu, for example, we can achieve our goals easily.

As it has been reiterated on several occasions, this type of food should be monitored by a nutritionist or expert in the area because each body reacts differently and the requirements of one person are not the ones of another person. In addition, each person may have different inflammatory problems or food allergy that should be considered before starting any diet. Although the keto diet is wonderful and has a wide variety of proven benefits, it is also true that each person should be evaluated by an expert.

CHAPTER 14:
BREAKFAST

When practicing a traditional eating plan (with this we mean one that has a normal intake of carbohydrates) it is said that breakfast is one of the most important meals of the day as people go a long period without eating food from the night of the last day. This implies that this is the first meal of the day; the one that allows people to get enough energy to face their day with all the challenges it can have. If you do not eat breakfast, and then eat lunch, for example, it is very likely that people will feel hungry throughout the day.

For the reasons stated above, it is important to show you some recipes in order to have a good ketogenic breakfast.

CUPS OF EGG, HAM, AND CHEESE

This is a very simple recipe, as you do not need many ingredients. They are cheese, ham, and eggs; these are ingredients that can be found in every fridge. Besides, this is not very complicated to prepare since you do not have to be a chef to make it. In addition, it can also be done very quickly, in an approximate time of twenty-five minutes. So, if you are in a hurry for the daily struggle, this recipe is very good for you. The ingredients are as follows:

- A spoonful of butter.
- Twelve slices of ham.
- A cup of shredded cheddar cheese, or a cheese that is fatty.
- Twelve large eggs.
- Salt to taste.
- Pepper to taste.
- Freshly chopped parsley.

When we see these ingredients, we can see that the recipe does not require anything out of the ordinary. Hence, anyone can make this recipe and as you will see below, it is not a very difficult process.

1. Preheat the oven at 400°.
2. Grease a tray of muffins with butter; you are going to grease the cavities of the muffins.
3. Place the slices of ham inside the muffin cavities covering them with the ham.

4. Place the cheese inside each cavity, above the ham that has already been placed.
5. Break one egg per muffin cavity on top of the cheese.
6. Season with pepper and salt to taste.
7. Decorate with parsley.

By observing how it is prepared, you can see that its preparation is extremely simple, for that reason, you can cook it without the need for having advanced knowledge in the kitchen. All you have to do is to preheat an oven, and then put ham, cheese, and egg; then wait until everything is ready. This recipe is very simple, but at the same time, it is very tasty.

STUFFED PEPPERS

For this recipe, not much is needed, only bell peppers and eggs. Obviously, you can add the ingredients you want, as long as what you want to add is allowed in the ketogenic diet. This recipe is as simple as the last one, but in this case, instead of using molds for muffins, we will be using the bell peppers.

The ingredients are as follows:

- Two large bell peppers, halved and seeded.
- Eight beaten eggs.
- A quarter of a cup of milk.
- Four strips of bacon, cooked and toasted, cut into small squares.
- One cup shredded cheddar cheese.
- Two tablespoons of scallions, finely chopped.
- Salt to taste.
- Pepper to taste.

As you could see, the recipe doesn't need many ingredients, and the ones you need are very common, therefore, for you to make this breakfast, you don't need many things. If that wasn't enough, the process to cook this breakfast is extremely simple.

1. Preheat the oven at 400°.
2. Place the peppers on a baking tray facing up and add a little water.
3. Put the peppers in the oven for about five minutes.
4. Beat the eggs and milk until smooth.
5. Add bacon pieces, cheese, spring onion, salt and pepper to taste.
6. Pour the mixture into the peppers, and leave them in the oven. Leave about thirty to forty minutes in the oven.

As you can see, this recipe is extremely simple and does not need much more than simple ingredients. This recipe consumes a little more time than the other one, but it is worth it, so we can only recommend you to cook it and try it.

CHAPTER 15:
LUNCH

Lunch is a vital meal for the human being, even despite being in a ketogenic diet, it is always important to eat three meals a day. Skipping one of the three main meals affects the metabolism of each person.

To be able to make such a diet, and not suffering in the attempt, we will recommend you to make the following recipes:

COBB EGG SALAD

Eating salad is always good, for that reason, we recommend you to eat it. It has different foods rich in fats; they are foods such as bacon or avocado that has natural fats which help our body to enter ketosis. The ingredients are as follows.

Ingredients:

- Three tablespoons of mayonnaise, preferably natural.
- Three spoonfuls of Greek yogurt, since it is the healthiest of all.
- Two spoonfuls of red wine.
- Kosher salt.
- Black pepper to taste, as this doesn't affect the ketosis process.
- Eight boiled eggs, you can chop as you wish, it is recommended to chop them into several round pieces for decoration, but if you are a person who does not care about the appearance, chop them as you like. That amount is the minimum, but you can use the amount of boiled eggs you want.
- Eight strips of bacon, which you can cut into strips or squares. At the time of cooking, this amount is recommended as a minimum, but you could consume more bacon, so you can decorate the Cobb egg salad.
- An avocado that should be cut into thin strips. You can cut it as you like either as squares or strips and you can consume the amount of avocado you wish.
- Half a cup of blue cheese shredded or crumbled, this the cheese is not exclusive, you can consume the cheese you want, such as smoked or yellow cheese as long as it is high in fat.
- Half a cup of cherry tomatoes, the same chopped in half. If you do not have this type of tomatoes, you can also eat regular tomatoes, chopped in small squares.

- A quantity of two tablespoons of chives chopped very small.

Now, the preparation process is very simple, only two simple steps are needed.

1. In a small bowl add the mayonnaise, the Greek yogurt, and the red wine, stir well until you have a homogeneous mixture, after having done that, proceed to add salt and pepper. This step is responsible for making the sauce, or rather the salad dressing.
2. Then, in a larger bowl, we proceed to add the eggs, bacon, cheese of your choice and cherry tomatoes; after they are all there we proceed to gradually add the dressing previously made, it is going to be added until all the ingredients are well covered with it, after that, try the salad and proceed to add salt and pepper to taste. Finally, add the chives to decorate the salad to taste.

As you could see, the process and the ingredients to make this salad were really very simple. The preparation should not take more than ten minutes since you only need to chop the vegetables, cook the bacon, make the eggs, and mix well, which should not take much time nor knowledge in the culinary field.

STUFFED AVOCADOS

This is a very simple and fast recipe, for which you do not need many ingredients. All you need are avocados, onions, fatty cheeses, nothing too exotic or very difficult to get because you only need things that you can get in your home market. Besides, you do not need to be a chef since this recipe is extremely simple; on the other hand, if you are in a hurry you won't waste a lot of time either since the time it will take you to prepare this recipe is between ten minutes or a little more. The recipe quantities are equivalent to about four portions for people who do not eat a lot, but for people who are used to eat a lot, could serve as two portions.

The ingredients are the following:

- Four avocados that are well ripe.
- The juice you can get from a lemon.
- A spoonful of olive oil, preferably extra virgin.
- An onion of medium size, which is chopped as you prefer.
- One pound of ground beef.
- Condiments of your preference to prepare the tacos. Moreover, there are packages made for you to prepare the tacos.
- Kosher salt to your liking.
- Black pepper, fresh and freshly ground.

- A cup of yellow cheese, or also Mexican shredded cheese.
- Half a cup of chopped lettuce.
- Small chopped cherry tomatoes, or regular tomatoes chopped in small squares.
- Sour cream, for consistency and decoration.

After having all these ingredients, we can proceed to the preparation but it should be noted that to make this recipe; the ingredients we just mentioned are the basic ones so if you want to add more ingredients you can do so. As long as you do not go out of what stipulates the ketogenic diet, which is not to consume carbohydrates or sugars. Well, explained that point, we will proceed to explain how to make its preparation.

1. We take our avocados and chop them in half, we take out the seed, boning the avocado, thus leaving as a hole in the avocado, which is the space occupied by the seed. Finally, we put lemon juice to our avocados, to prevent them from oxidizing.
2. Then, place in a frying pan over medium heat the oil until it is bubbly, at that time, that the oil is very hot, add the onions that had already been chopped. Let them cook until they are golden, this may take a little bit, about three or five minutes.
3. Add the ground beef and the seasoning of your preference; then, with the help of a wooden spoon, move the meat, also keep seasoning with salt and pepper. Afterward, the beef is going to be put together in the pan with the onions. Cook until the meat is not pink, this meat cooking lasts about five or six minutes.
4. After the meat is cooked, drain the fat from it.
5. After draining the meat, proceed to grab the avocado and fill in the avocado holes with all seasoned ground beef. Finally, at the top of the stuffed avocado, add the cheese, tomato, lettuce, sour cream and enjoy your meal.

As you could see, in order to make the avocado tacos recipe you don't need to be a chef. It only takes a little time, and it's not much since it should take about ten minutes, therefore, this recipe is extremely effective when you are busy or in a hurry. Besides, it will allow you to continue with a keto lifestyle without losing or skipping good meals because practicing this style of food, does not mean eating badly or insipid, it is quite the opposite.

KETO BACON SUSHI

For lovers of Asian food, especially those of sushi, we have this dish, which is not really sushi but it has its form because when preparing it, we will give it the shape of them. It is very similar to the traditional sushi, but a ketogenic one. No special ingredients are needed either, because you can use carrots, bell peppers, among others. It is also important to say that this recipe will also provide a perfect balance, as you will eat vegetables and some fats. The estimated time to make this recipe, adding the time to chop all the ingredients, and then cook them, is half an hour, therefore, although we could see an increase in time when cooking the recipe, we can also see that we are expanding our menu with simple recipes.

The ingredients are as follows:

- Six slices of bacon, the same chopped in half, to then be able to use them to make the covering of the pieces of sushi. The bacon in this recipe will act as the seaweed, which will cover the sushi.
- Two cucumbers, it is recommended that the same are chopped into thin slices.
- Two medium carrots, it is also recommended that the carrots are chopped into very thin slices.
- Four ounces of cream cheese, quite soft, so that after it can be mixed with other things.
- Sesame seeds to decorate.

After having the ingredients chopped and everything ready, we proceed to begin the cooking process, but not before specifying that we can make keto sushi with any vegetable, in this case, we are using carrots, but they can be replaced by bell peppers to say something different than carrots. Now, let's get to work.

1. The first step is to preheat the oven to four hundred Celsius degrees.
2. We take some of our trays, which we use for baking and we will wrap it in aluminum foil.
3. Place the bacon on top of the aluminum that has covered your tray, so that it can be cooked. It must be placed in such a way that the halves of the bacon are in a symmetrical way or better said, place the bacon so as to create a uniform layer. They should be baked until the bacon is crispy but also that a little easy to fold, possessing a certain grade of flexibility.
4. Then cut the carrots, avocados, and cucumbers to the same width as the bacon.
5. After the bacon has rested so that you can touch them with your hands, you will proceed to put a little cream cheese on top of the ends of the bacon and proceed to take the vegetables that you had already chopped and place them evenly on it. Preferably, place those vegetables at the ends of the bacon.
6. Roll up the vegetables quickly and tightly with the bacon.
7. Finally, we proceeded to decorate the recipe with seeds of alamo to the taste of each guest.

As we could see with this recipe, which sounds delicious, you don't need a lot to eat delicious, you just need imagination and a little time. As we said previously, vegetables can be replaced, not only we can make keto sushi with carrots, we can also use tomatoes, bell peppers, cucumbers, among other foods. You just need imagination to make this recipe more diverse and more delicious.

As you could see in this chapter, with these three recipes of ketogenic lunches, you will not lose the quality of your food, only that you will not consume carbohydrates. With this, we mean that your food will not lose flavor. Instead, it will maintain it, therefore, you will not find it difficult to migrate to this type of ketogenic food since as you can imagine, the flavor is delicious and you will be feeding better, cellularly speaking. What we can tell you is to try these recipes, investigate new and different recipes to make variated lunches, and create your own ones.

CHAPTER 16:
DINNERS

Generally, dinner is a dish that is difficult to plan. Perhaps we spend all day in most cases in the street and when we get home we do not want very elaborated or difficult menus. Nevertheless, there will be special occasions in which we will have time to prepare a delicious dinner. For those who practice fasting, probably this is their second meal of the day, for those who don't, we talk about the third meal of the day. Regardless of the case, we must take into account that at the evening meal it is recommended not to consume or reduce to the maximum the consumption of carbohydrates. In this order of ideas, we will give some recipes for dinner following the ketogenic style.

BREASTS STUFFED WITH PESTO SAUCE AND MOZZARELLA CHEESE

Ingredients:

- 3 breasts
- 250 grams of Mozzarella cheese approximately, if you like a lot of cheese add more.
- A large fresh bunch of basil.
- 1 clove of garlic
- Olive oil to taste
- A handful of almonds
- Shredded Parmesan cheese to taste.
- Salt and pepper to taste

Steps to Follow:

1. Wash the basil leaves well and add them to the glass of the blender. Now add the almonds and the whole peeled clove of garlic. Then add 3 to 4 tablespoons of olive oil, a little salt, and pepper to taste and proceed to blend. We must obtain a creamy emulsion; if we see that it lacks more liquid, we can add more oil until it reaches the point that more pleases us to the palate.
2. We must ensure that everything (especially the garlic) is well crushed.
3. When the sauce is ready, blended, and with the desired consistency, add the Parmesan cheese and, if you want, blend again at medium speed, there are people who do not blend the cheese and can do so as well.

4. Now with this delicious pesto, we are going to fill the breasts.
5. We are going to open the breasts like books, and we are going to add salt and pepper to taste.
6. We add a good and appetizing layer of the pesto we already prepared and later we place several slices of Mozzarella cheese on top.
7. Roll up the breasts and hold them with sticks of wood or bamboo.
8. We can cook them in the oven or in a non-stick frying pan. And the tasty dinner of breasts stuffed with pesto and Parmesan cheese is ready.

HAKE WITH ROMESCO SAUCE AND VEGETABLES

This dish is ideal for the night when you want to make a more elaborate meal. The sauce is ideal to accompany both fish and chicken as the case may be. This recipe is designed to get a thick sauce, you can make it more liquid if you like. Here I use the hake but you can choose the fish you want.

Ingredients:

- 1 ¼ Cup of Almonds
- 2 cloves garlic
- 500 grams of bell peppers
- 3 Tomatoes
- 1 Gren onion
- Half Onion or a medium Onion.
- Olive Oil
- Salt to taste
- Pepper to taste
- 3 Hake

Steps to follow:

1. First, let's make the sauce. Cut the bell peppers into pieces and process them together with the tomato, onion, garlic, and almonds; you have to process them very. We are going to process for about 30 seconds; when we are processing everything we add about three or four tablespoons of olive oil. We see the consistency as we process the mixture. When we say process we mean to cook.
2. When the sauce is ready we proceed to make the hake, once cleaned and filleted we add a little lemon, this step is optional according to the taste of each one, but the seasoning with lemon gives a wonderful aroma and flavor to the fish. Then we are going to season

with salt and pepper. And we are going to place them in a frying pan, preferably non-stick, and cook carefully over medium heat until they are ready. Obviously, we will have to turn them so that they cook on both sides.

3. Once ready and served, add the romesco sauce on top of the hake.

If you wish, you can accompany it with avocado and stir-fried bacon, it is a wonderful combination for this dish.

BROCCOLI AND SAUSAGE TORTILLA

It is a simple dish to make for dinner and within the standards of the ketogenic diet. If you like it you can add more vegetables to it.

Ingredients:

- 1 large whole broccoli.
- 2 or 3 sausages; should be organic chicken, preferably pre-cooked.
- Clarified Butter or Ghee.
- 6 large eggs preferably.
- Fresh oregano, chopped parsley.
- Salt to taste.
- Pepper to taste.
- 1 avocado.

Steps to follow.

1. The first thing we are going to do is to cook the broccoli. It is recommended to boil the water first in a pot and once the water is boiling we are going to place the broccoli in a period of about 3 to 5 minutes since we do not want it to be overcooked. Actually, it will be better al dente. Once cooked the broccoli, we submerge it in ice water to stop the cooking, and later we chop it in small pieces and add salt to taste.
2. In a frying pan add ghee butter and the sausages that were previously thinly sliced and cook them. When they are ready, add the broccoli, fry it together with the sausages and add salt, oregano, finely chopped parsley to taste, and fry it a few more minutes. In a bowl, we are going to pour the eggs and beat them until obtaining a homogeneous mixture.
3. Then in the pan where we have the sausage and broccoli fried, we are going to pour the eggs and let them cook for a few minutes. When we observe that the tortilla is almost

done, we remove it carefully from the pan, we take it off and turn it so that it is cooked on the other side for a few more minutes.

4. Once the tortilla is ready we serve it and on top of it, we are going to put the sliced avocado, in addition, if it is of our taste we can sprinkle over it a little salt and pepper to give the final touch.

CHAPTER 17:
SWEET TOOTHS, SNACKS AND DESSERTS

When starting any diet and mainly the Keto diet, we could feel hungry or anxious at some moments. To avoid that feeling it is advisable to eat some snacks as long as they are carbohydrates-free. This way we can stay in the Keto line.

Let's remember that snacks are mostly a type of light food that we eat when we have anxiety, these in a certain way give us energy. The problem occurs when these snacks are eaten in large quantities and very often, as they are made from heavy ingredients that provide more fat to our body.

There are many ways to calm the anxiety or feeling of hunger with pleasant and healthy options so that we have are not guilty of giving us a taste. Next, we are going to show you a variety of options of snacks approved by experts in keto that will keep us satisfied without leaving the diet.

These recipes could be ideal as a snack or even as a dinner since they do not require much preparation:

- Slice of cheese spread with butter
- Celery stuffed with cream cheese
- Slice of cold butter spread with peanut butter
- Lettuce or cucumber spread with mayonnaise
- Small radishes with butter
- Parmesan cheese fries with butter
- Cheese and salami slices rolled up
- Sliced bacon with peanut butter or butter
- A square of dark chocolate with butter
- One tablespoon of butter or coconut oil melted in tea or coffee

On the other hand, we have a list of snacks a little more elaborated and tasty for those moments of anxiety. Ketogenic snacks are a good option to keep us on the diet in case we feel hungry.

EGGPLANT FRENCH FRIES

Ingredients:

- 2 eggplants
- 475 ml (250 g) ground almonds
- 1 tsp cayenne pepper
- Salt and black pepper to taste
- 2 eggs
- 2 tbsp. coconut oil spray

Preparation:

1. Preheat oven to 400°F (200°C).
2. Peel the eggplants and cut into chips. Add salt (a little) on all sides to prevent the eggplant from becoming bitter.
3. In a not very deep bowl, mix the ground almond, cayenne, and pepper, in another bowl add the eggs beating until frothy.
4. Pass the chopped eggplants through the almonds, through the eggs and again through the almonds.
5. Place the eggplants "potatoes" in a baking tray previously greased, sprinkle coconut oil on top.
6. Bake for 15 minutes or until golden brown and crispy.

BACON AND CHEDDAR CHEESE BALLS

These balls are not only delicious but also ketogenic, bacon and cheddar cheese are a perfect and delicious combination, here we leave the preparation:

Ingredients:

- 150 g bacon
- 1 tablespoon of butter
- 150 g (150 ml) cream cheese
- 150 g cheddar cheese
- 50 g butter (at room temperature)
- ½ tsp ground black pepper

Preparation:

1. Melt the butter and fry the bacon until golden brown.
2. Remove from the frying pan and let cool on absorbent paper.
3. Cut the bacon into small pieces and place them in a bowl.
4. In another bowl, mix the excess fat from the bacon with the rest of the ingredients.

5. Leave the mixture in the refrigerator for 15 minutes to harden the mixture.
6. Assemble the balls, pass them over the bacon and serve.

SPINACH, ARTICHOKE AND CREAM CHEESE DIP

Ingredients:

- 1 cucumber, chopped into sticks
- 2 cups spinach
- 2 artichoke hearts
- 1 tsp cream cheese
- Grain salt

Preparation:

1. Cook the spinach with a little grain salt, drain and cool.
2. Chop the cucumbers and reserve
3. Chop the artichoke hearts into four, add them in a bowl with the spinach.
4. Add the cream cheese, seasoning and mixing everything.

FOCACCIA BREAD WITH GARLIC AND ROSEMARY

Ingredients:

- 175 g (375 m) shredded mozzarella.
- 2 tbsp (30g) cream cheese.
- 1 tsp. white wine vinegar.
- 1 egg.
- 175 ml (100 g) ground almonds.
- ½ tsp of salt.
- ½ tsp garlic powder.
- 50 g butter at room temperature.
- 3 cloves garlic, finely chopped
- ½ teaspoon of sea salt
- ½ tsp fresh chopped rosemary

Preparation:

1. Preheat oven to 200 °C (400 °F)

2. Heat cream cheese and mozzarella cheese in a saucepan over medium heat (microwaves can also be used) and stir occasionally.
3. Add the rest of the ingredients and mix.
4. Flatten the dough to a round shape, no more than 20 cm above the baking paper.
5. Using a fork, make small holes, bake for 12 minutes or until golden brown, then remove and let cool.
6. Prepare a mixture with garlic, butter, salt and rosemary, spread on bread and place on a grill or grill
7. Leave for 7 minutes

MEXICAN-STYLE SAUSAGES

Ingredients:

- ½ cup chopped onion
- ½ tomato
- 2 turkey sausages
- Chili
- Grain salt

Preparation:

1. Add onion in a pan over medium heat until translucent.
2. Add the chili together with the tomato chopped in cubes, season with salt.
3. Chop the sausages in slices and add the sauce, let cook and serve.

LETTUCE CUBES WITH PRICKLY PEAR SALAD

Ingredients:

- Lettuce (4 firm leaves well washed)
- 2 prickly pears
- Grain salt
- ½ cup onion
- 1 tsp olive oil
- 1 tsp vinegar
- 1 tbsp. chopped coriander
- 1 small chili-tomato

Preparation:

1. In a refractory add the prickly pears in cubes and leave them overnight with salt in grain (well covered).
2. Next day drain and let dry
3. Cut the onion and tomato into cubes and add them to the nopales.
4. Add olive oil, chopped coriander, and vinegar.
5. Place the mixture on the lettuce

PREPARED OLIVES

Ingredients:

- 1 lemon (juice)
- ¼ cup chopped onion
- 6 Kalamata olives, pitted and stuffed
- 2 tbsp soy sauce

Preparation:

1. Cook the onion in a frying pan until translucent.
2. Add the olives and sprinkle with the sauce and lemon.
3. Let cool and serve

CAULIFLOWER BITS WITH PEANUT BUTTER

Ingredients:

- 2 tbsp peanut butter
- coarse salt
- 1 tbsp olive oil
- 1 cauliflower

Preparation:

1. Preheat oven to 400°F (200°C)
2. Cut the cauliflower
3. On a tray with waxed paper, put the cauliflowers and add olive oil, season and bake until golden brown.
4. Remove from oven and spread peanut butter, bake for a couple more minutes.

5. Remove from oven, let cool and serve

Additionally, for those who need something fast due to their short time due to work or travel, there are adequate snacks to the keto diet, among the most prominent are:

- Packaged olives (green, black or assorted)
- Beef bar (shredded pork or chicken sriracha)
- Cooked bacon
- Salami snacks
- Pork cracklings
- Macadamia nuts
- Pili nuts
- Very dark chocolate

CHARD SKEWERS WITH HAM AND CHEESE

Ingredients:

- 3 thin slices of cooked ham
- 3 thin slices of cheese
- 3 leaves of chard well cleaned
- 2 large tomatoes, well washed

Preparation:

Cook the chard for a maximum time of 2 minutes, take it out of the water and then let it cool until it can be manipulated. Then, place it on a tray or plate and put on it the slices of ham and cheese carefully to avoid breaking the chards and roll them up. We chop in rolls and we take out three portions to assemble the skewer placing in each end a cube of tomato, then to serve. This recipe of skewers is perfect to consume between meals as a salty snack, however for the one that prefers, it can be a recipe for a dinner rich in proteins.

CRACKERS OF CRUNCHY SEEDS AND OATS

Ingredients:

- 20 grams of poppy seeds
- 20 grams of linseed
- 25 grams of chia seeds

- 55 grams of sesame seed
- 55 grams of pumpkin seeds
- 20 grams of thin layers of oats
- ¼ of caraway seeds
- ¼ teaspoon of granulated garlic or a clove of grated garlic
- 250ml of water

Preparation:

Turn on the oven at 150°C, place all the ingredients in a container except for the water, mix them all very well, add the water stirring little by little until it integrates with all the ingredients, leave to rest well covered for 10 minutes. After the time has elapsed, check that the water has been absorbed by the seeds. Its consistency should be a sticky dough where not even a drop should be left, otherwise, add a little oatmeal or chia, mix and wait again.

Place in the tray greased paper and then flatten using a roller or a kitchen spatula, the mixture should not be more than 3 to 5mm thick, put in the oven for a time of 30 to 35 minutes. After that time, with the spatula, introduce underneath the mixture, trying to turn very carefully to prevent it from breaking (you can use board or large plate), bake again for 25 to 30 minutes more, be careful to avoid burning. Remove from the oven, wait for it to cool down, cut on a board and cut with a good knife into pieces.

CHAPTER 18: KETO DRINKS

As well as the Keto diet offers us varieties in sweet tooths and snacks to be consumed without any remorse, it also provides us different drinks and

smoothies that are allowed and are within the ketogenic standards. Here we show you the different options so that you can choose according to your preference:

KETO SMOOTHIE CHOCOLATE

Have a necessary quantity of zucchini, coconut milk, and lettuce at your disposal. Romana, chia seeds, spinach, cocoa powder, avocado, sweetener of

Passion fruit and mix everything to obtain a rich and sweet drink.

Chia seeds with blueberries and coconut

- 1 cup cashew or almond milk
- 2 tbsp. coconut oil
- 2 tbsp. ground chia seeds
- Sweetener equivalent to 2 tablespoons of sugar
- 1 cup blueberries
- 1 cup Greek yogurt (can be substituted for coconut milk without milk)
- ½ cup coconut

Mix all ingredients

SMOOTHIE FOR BREAKFAST

It is a rich cocktail ideal to start the day based on the following ingredients: Spinach, coconut milk, greens powder, whey protein, almonds, Brazil nuts, spinach, sweet potato starch, and psyllium seeds; optionally, you can add some almonds to give a greater nutty flavor, then mix all the ingredients together and you'll get a nutritious drink to start the day.

Green shake

You only need the necessary amount of lemon, cucumber, avocado, and kale, all this is mixed with water, then blended and ready, is a rich and healthy drink

Smoothie with almond milk

This drink apart from being rich and healthy provides nutrients needed to start the day, you will only need celery, cucumber, matcha, spinach, avocado, and almond milk, then mix all the ingredients and finally, we add the chia seeds and coconut oil

Chia shake

This drink provides us with fiber

Ingredients:

- 1 tbsp walnut butter
- 1 tablespoon of chia seeds (soaked in water for 10 minutes)
- ¼ cup coconut milk
- 1 avocado
- 2 tsp. cocoa beans (if you want to add more flavor)
- 1 tsp. cocoa powder
- 1 scoop of chocolate protein powder
- 1 tbsp coconut oil

Blend all the ingredients mixing uniformly. If it is too thick, you can add 1 cup of water. At the moment of serving you can decorate with cocoa beans and cinnamon.

Green milkshake (without dairy products)

It is called green milkshake because it is the predominant color, the ingredients to use are avocado, kiwi, fresh ginger, fresh parsley, raw cucumber, fresh pineapple, and lettuce. We blend all the ingredients with water and we sweeten with any sugar substitute that is to your liking and preference.

Smoothie with macadamia nut oil

To prepare this shake you only need to mix avocado, spinach, stevia, coconut milk, cream, macadamia nut oil, vanilla protein, and oil of avocado, if you don't want to add or you don't have avocado oil at your disposal it can be replaced by olive oil or peanut oil.

Milkshake of almonds and blueberries

What it is necessary to achieve this tasty and nutrient-rich drink is to combine sugar-free almond sugar, a small amount of blueberries preferably organic, almond butter (it must be raw) and MCT oil

Strawberry milkshake

To achieve an excellent blend and obtain this smoothie it is necessary:

- 1 cup of fresh strawberries
- 1 tsp vanilla extract
- 1 tbsp coconut oil (you can also use any other healthy oil)
- 450ml coconut milk, if not available can be replaced by a cup of Greek yogurt if you prefer a milkshake (add water if it's too thick).

Raspberry vanilla smoothie

Ingredients:

- ½ cup natural strawberries (can be frozen)
- ½ cup unsweetened coconut milk
- 2/3 cup water
- ½ vanilla tsp (extract)

Then mix all the ingredients in the blender

Beet Smoothie

Mix in the blender the following ingredients to enjoy a delicious smoothie.

- 1 tbsp coconut oil
- 1 tbsp whey protein
- 1 tsp powdered cinnamon
- 1 cup almond milk, coconut milk can also be used
- 1 tbsp powdered beet

Walnut Smoothie:

- 1 pinch of salt
- 1 tsp powdered cinnamon
- 1 tablespoon peanut butter or cashew butter
- 2 tbsp preferably ground flax seeds
- 2 tbsp peeled walnuts
- 1 cup almonds

Combine all ingredients and blend

Ginger Smoothie

- Ingredients for its preparation:
- 30g frozen spinach
- 2 tbsp lemon juice
- 150ml of water
- 2 tsp. fresh stuffed ginger
- 75ml coconut cream or coconut milk

Combine all ingredients, add tablespoons of lemon one at a time. one to achieve the desired taste, after serving the drink we add a little of grated ginger and sprinkle over it.

Ketogenic coffee with cinnamon

This drink is ideal for those cold days, to make it you will need the following ingredients:

- 1 tsp ground cinnamon
- 475ml of water
- 2 tbsp ground coffee
- 75ml whipping cream

We combine the coffee with the cinnamon. We add the water and make it like coffee is normally made. Beat the cream with the help of a mixer until you get a mixture to point of snow, we serve in a large cup the coffee, add the whipped cream over it and finally add the cinnamon.

Chai tea

It is a warm and aromatic drink perfect for cold and rainy days.

Ingredients:

- 475ml of water
- 75ml whipping cream
- 1 tbsp chai tea

Follow the instructions on the chai tea container (hot water and tea), in the microwave, heat the cream in a medium cup and add the tea.

Coffee with pumpkinspices

Ingredients:

- ½ Tbsp vanilla extract
- 1 tbsp (25g) erythritol
- 1 tsp. spice mix for pumpkin pie
- 60ml (60g) pumpkin puree
- 60ml decaffeinated espresso coffee can also be strong coffee
- 225ml hot, unsweetened almond milk

Preparation:

Add all the ingredients in a blender and blend until a soft mixture is obtained, try it and give it the taste according to your preference, finally serve it.

Eggnog

Ingredients:

- ¼ honey tsp
- 1 pinch of ground nutmeg
- 225ml whipping cream
- 1 orange, the zest, and the juice
- 4 tbsp. brandy or any dark liqueur
- ¼ Tbsp vanilla extract

Preperation:

1. Mix the honey, vanilla powder and beaten egg yolks until the mixture is smooth, add ¼ of orange. Then we add 4 tablespoons of juice of orange, with the liqueur, carefully mix the whipping cream and combine it in a bowl with the egg mixture.
2. Serve in glasses and take to the refrigerator for 15 minutes.
3. This helps to develop more flavor and consistency in the eggnog

Flavored water

The cold flavored water refreshes when we feel like something without the need of adding calories Ingredients:

- 1 liter of cold, freshwater
- Flavorings of your free choice that can be fresh mint, cucumber or raspberries
- 475ml of ice

Preparation

1- Add the cold water in a pitcher

2- Place the chosen flavor and take it to the refrigerator leaving it to rest for at least 30 minutes
3- Fresh mint, citrus fruits such as orange, lemon or berries can be added if desired
4- With only a few slices are enough to give a rich flavor

Cold coffee

To soothe the heat, this delicious iced drink is an excellent choice.

Ingredients:

- 60ml whipping cream
- 225ml of coffee
- Ice cubes
- Vanilla extract (optional)

Instructions

1- As usual prepare the coffee, but twice as usual and leave it to cool down.
2- In a large glass add the ice cubes, add the coffee and then the cream.
3- Serve

Coffee with ketogenic cream

Ingredients:

- 60ml whipping cream
- 180ml of coffee

Preparation:

1- Choose the coffee of your preference and prepare it as usual.
2- In a small pot add the cream and heat, stir gently until it becomes frothy
3- In a large cup, pour the hot cream, add the coffee and stir
4- Serve instantly accompanied by a handful of yummy walnuts.

Keto Cheesecake

Ingredients:

- 2 passion fruit
- 2 tablespoons ricotta cheese
- 1 sachet of stevia

- 1 glass almond milk
- ice to taste

Preparation:

Add all the ingredients in a blender, mix everything and you're done. This way we'll get a delicious drink.

CHAPTER 19: 7 DAY MEAL PLAN:

The 7-day meal plan aims to give a general idea of how the ketogenic diet might work effectively, however it is important to remember that it may work differently in each body.

This plan is based on a diet high in fat, low in carbohydrates and moderate in protein on which we could base the first week of our keto diet, however, we can refer to previous chapters for more recipes.

MONDAY

Breakfast: 2 sausages rolled in turkey with feta cheese and green tea

Snack: keto chocolate cheesecake

Lunch: Chicken Salad

Snack: pork rinds

Dinner: steamed vegetables and salmon

TUESDAY

Breakfast: Cheese and mushroom omelet

Snack: Coffee without sugar

Lunch: Mexican Chicken Tacos

Snack: squares of ham and cheese

Dinner: Shrimp brochettes with bacon and onion

WEDNESDAY

Breakfast: 2 boiled eggs wrapped in bacon strips and avocado strips

with green tea

Snack: Light gelatin

Lunch: Chicken breast stuffed with ham and cream cheese.

Snack: Celery sticks with guacamole

Dinner: chop suey

THURSDAY

Breakfast: Turkey sausage and blended protein with strawberries

Snack: 40 grams of peanuts

Lunch: Steamed broccoli with fish

Snack: Nuts

Dinner: Fish skewers with bell pepper

FRIDAY

Breakfast: Keto waffles with egg, cheese, and bacon

Snack: Coffee

Lunch: Asian-style sauteed keto cabbage

snack: gelatine

dinner: ham and cheese rolls

SATURDAY

Breakfast: salmon and bell pepper omelet

Snack: Merey

Lunch: Keto Caprese Omelet

Snack: Keto Smoothie

Dinner: Beef wraps

SUNDAY

Breakfast: Low-carbohydrate banana waffles

Snack: keto chocolate cake

Lunch: Ketogenic Tex Mex Casserole

Snack: Coconut biscuits without oven

Dinner: Stuffed avocados with smoked salmon

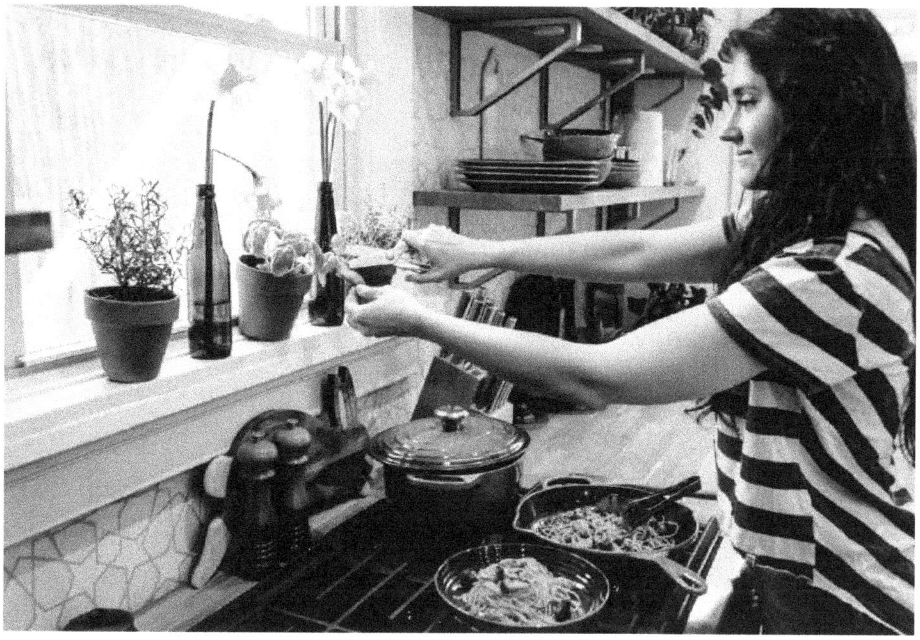

CONCLUSION

Thank you for making it through to the end of Keto for women: The ultimate beginners guide to know your food needs, weight loss, diabetes prevention and boundless energy with high-fat ketogenic diet recipes, let's hope it was informative and able to provide you with all of the tools you need to achieve your goals whatever they may be.

Now that you made it to the end of the book, you may know some, not to say all, of the benefits that the keto diet will have in your body. Even though it may be really hard to get started into this feeding plan, it absolutely worth it. Do not give up, fight for what you want, learn what your body needs and give it to it.

Women are known for being brave, amazing fighters and really strong so, are you going to let some extra pounds turn you down? As you could read, this diet is not only made for losing weight, there are studies that prove that this diet helps people who suffer from diabetes, decreases the symptoms of POS, helps in menstruation problems, improves brain and many other organs of our body.

Please, remember that even if you understood everything that is written in this book, and you feel like you can go keto on your own, it really recommended to go with a nutritionist or a specialist in the area for what you are using keto diet for. For example, if you are using keto to control POS, visit first your gyno.

Finally, if you found this book useful in any way, a review on Amazon is always appreciated!

Keto And Intermittent Fasting

Your Essential Guide for a Low-Carb Diet for Perfect Mind-Body Balance, Weight Loss, With Ketogenic Recipes to Maxizime Your Health

By

Kyndra Backer

INTRODUCTION

Congratulations on purchasing Keto and intermittent fasting: Your Essential Guide for a Low-Carb Diet for Perfect Mind-Body Balance, Weight Loss, With Ketogenic Recipes to Maximize Your Health and thank you for doing so.

We really hope that you are able to get the most benefit of this book since it was made with a lot of effort and willingness to help people to improve their health, lose weight or overcome any of the problems that the keto diet can help with.

In the following chapters, you will be able to find tons of really interesting information, starting from scratch, about the keto diet, how it works, benefits, risks, fasting, autophagy, how to relate both keto and intermittent fasting and many other awesome facts that will help you to change your lifestyle, starting from your feeding habits.

The chapters here written will teach you everything you need to know about the Ketogenic diet, the state of ketosis, which foods are allowed when following keto diet, fasting and different types of fasting, how to know if I am able to stick to this diet, why does people stress and how will this diet help about it, mental improvements, and many many other extraordinary information.

There are plenty of books on this subject on the market, thanks again for choosing this one! Every effort was made to ensure it is full of as much useful information as possible; please enjoy!

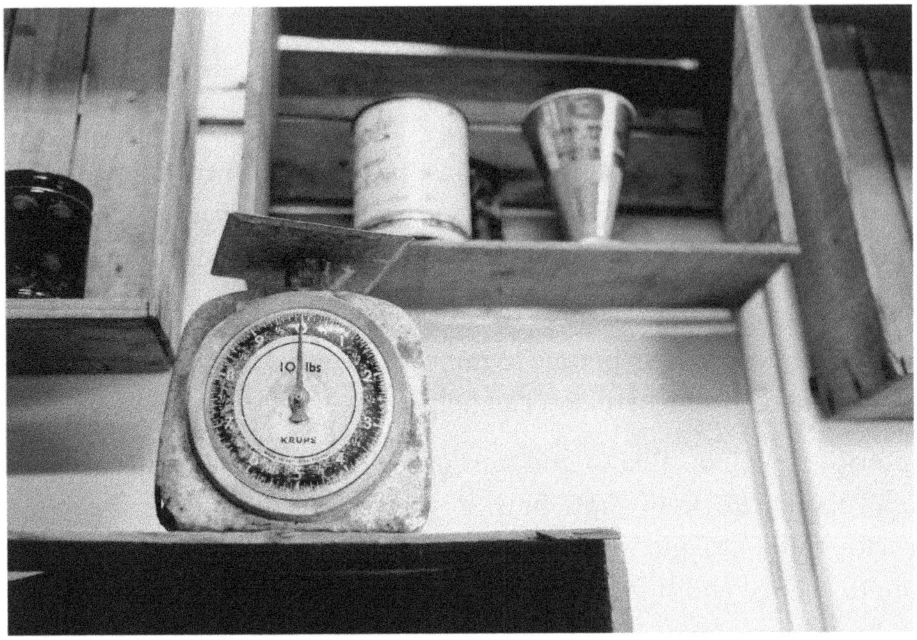
10 lbs
KRUPS

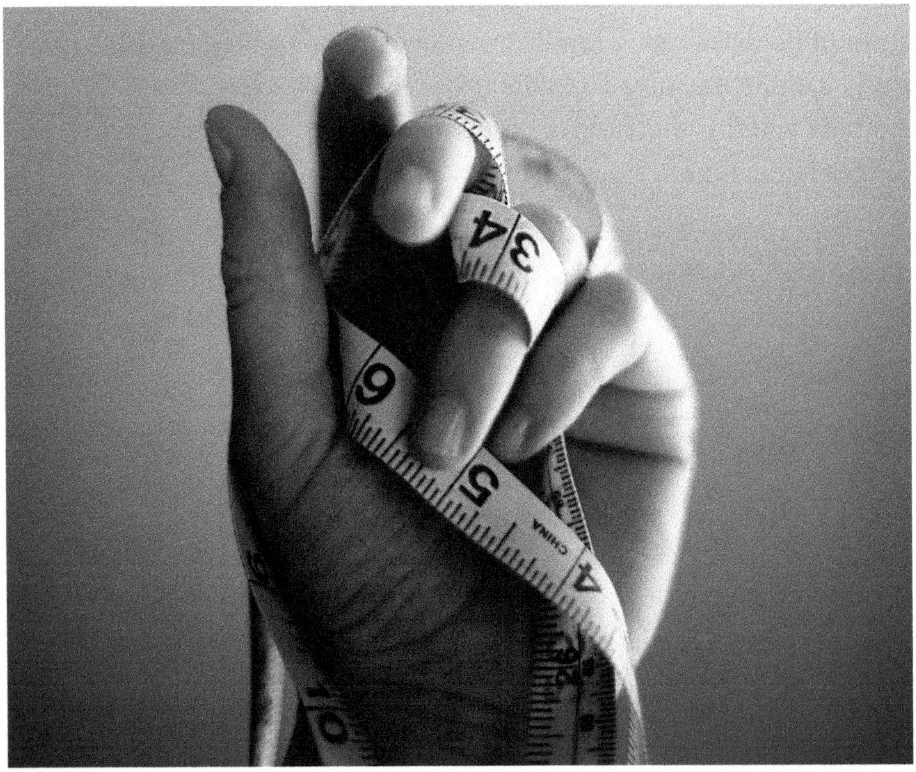
CHINA

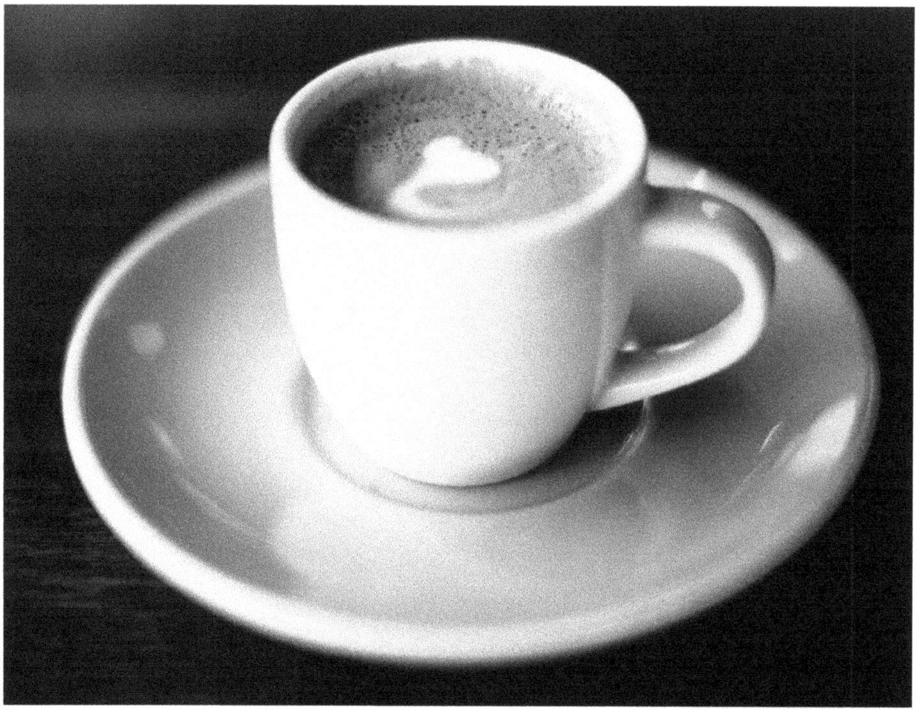

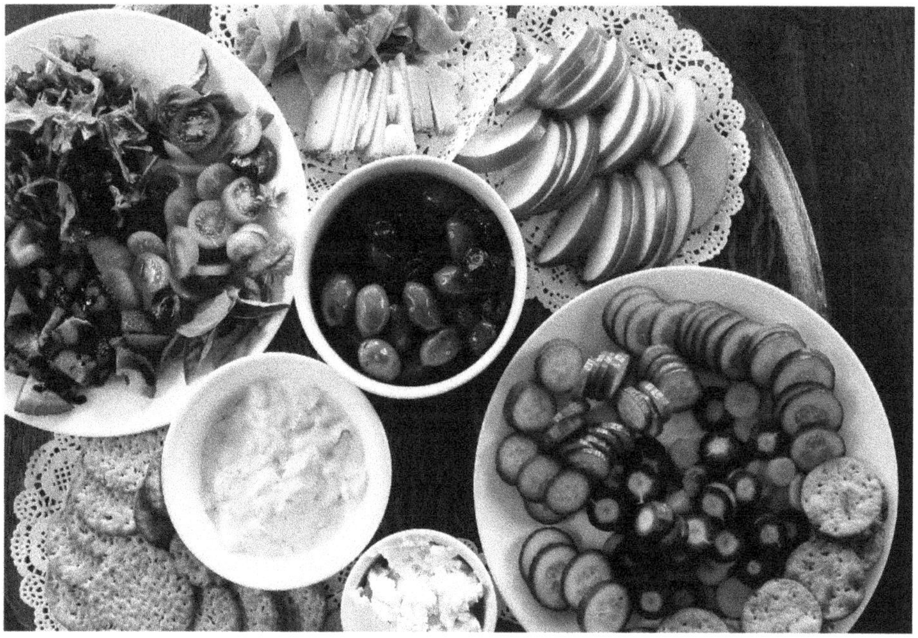

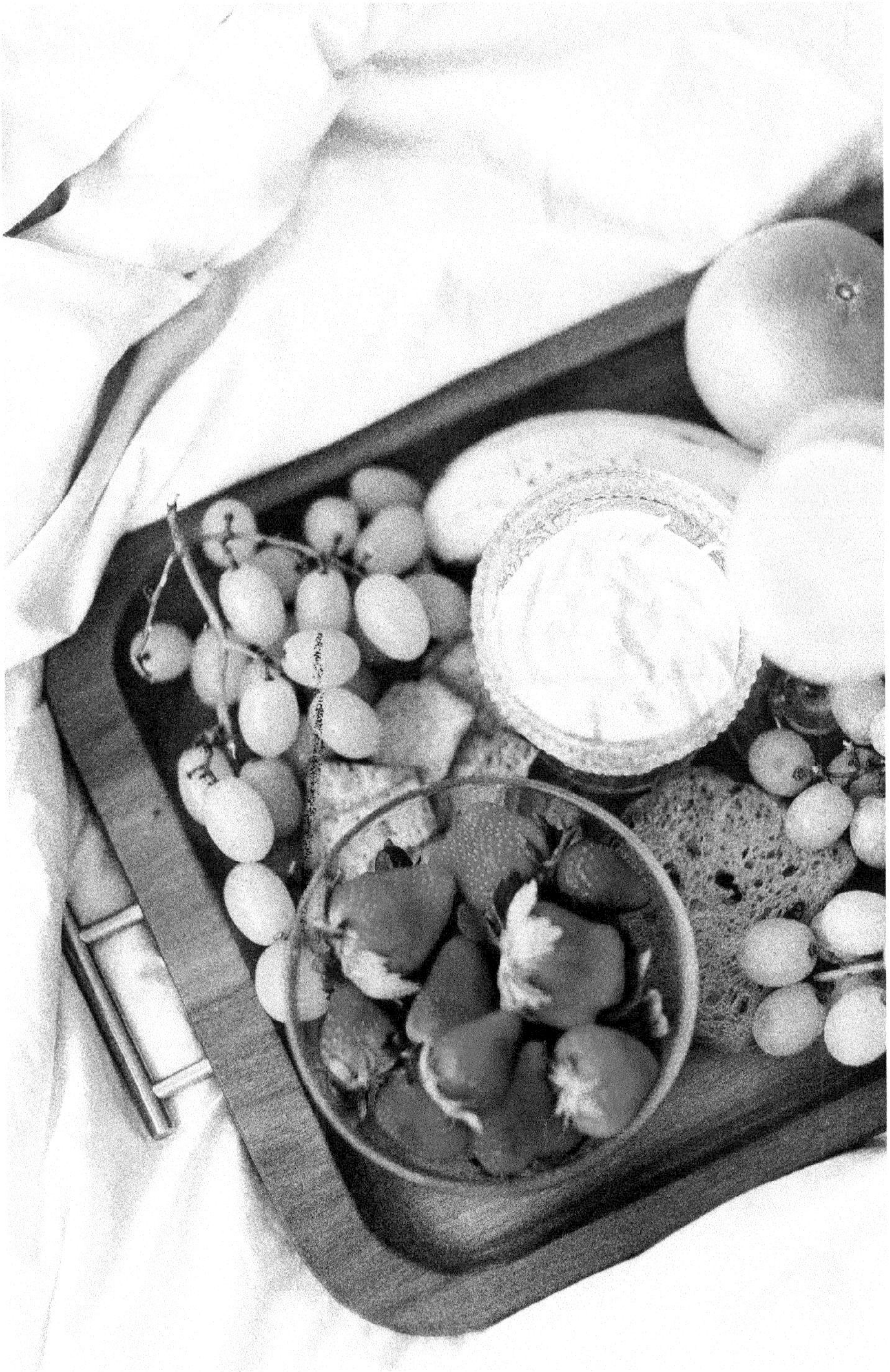

CHAPTER 1: WHAT IS THE KETOGENIC DIET?

Possibly when we hear about the word diet, the erroneous idea of restricting the free consumption of food and limiting ourselves to only a few nutrients and energies which are considered "necessary" in order to lose weight comes to mind.

Before going into the subject of what could be the ketogenic diet, let's define some concepts, which will be very helpful and supportive for the following chapters.

What does the word Diet mean? This word whose meaning is "regime of life" comes from the Greek word "dayta," this refers to the consumption of food that we do in our day to day (each one with a lapse of 24 hours) to our organism.

With the passing of the years the word diet has acquired much power and importance in the daily life of the human being, whether by leading a good lifestyle, a belief or simply curiosity; currently there are millions of characteristics associated with this word (this could be: low sodium diet, vegetarian diet, reduction diet, keto diet) the important thing is that you must always meet the following characteristics so that it can be called this way, a "diet":

It must be complete; a properly balanced diet must include all the nutrients necessary to provide all those vitamins and minerals that our body needs.

A diet should not imply a risk to our health, just as there are abundant foods in nutrients, there are foods that contain toxins and pollutants for our body, and these must be consumed with much moderation.

At the moment of ingesting the food, our plate must be proportionally balanced (there should not be more nutrients than others, it is suggested that all are the same).

The plate of our food to ingest must cover the sufficient nutrients that we need to have a correct weight. (and in the case of children, good growth and correct development.) It is never advisable to overload our dishes with nutrients to be completely full because being satisfied helps our body a lot.

A correct diet must be varied; it is advisable to include different types of nutrients in each group or portion.

And finally the most important because, to be able to eat well, we have to feel comfortable, our food must be according to our personal taste, this can also influence our culture, economic resources or any other factor.

It is very important to keep in mind that each diet is personalized because each person does not have the same physical condition, depending on this will reflect their mood, physical energy, mental capacity, body humor, physical aspects such as skin, hair, body odors and even health.

Up to this point, we must surely be asking ourselves, How can I start a correct diet if I have led a disordered lifestyle (in terms of my diet)?

To be able to "start" or just eat properly, we must be strong and put aside those treats, reduce certain foods that harm us; these could be: heavy flours, certain cereals, sugary foods, and many other foods that we are used to eating. And the most important thing: it is not to eat less, it is to increase the number of meals per day diminishing the portions in each plate; in this way, we are balancing our organism.

One way to clearly see the example of what a diet is is the ketogenic diet, which is well known for being a low-carbohydrate diet, which helps us burn fat more effectively.

By ingesting carbohydrates, our body produces substances such as glucose and insulin, which our body needs in order to produce energy. Both substances work together within our bloodstream.

MEANING OF KETO

The ketogenic diet was developed at the beginning of the 20th century by doctors, who were looking for a diet based on high-fat consumption, in order to control seizures in children. It had long been observed that fasting worked as a kind of treatment for epilepsy but of course, it was not possible for a person to fast for the rest of his life, which is why they began to use this type of food in epileptic patients where their diet was going to be based on the highest consumption of fat.

Over time it was observed that these patients who had followed the ketogenic style of feeding had decreased their seizures and even in a minority had disappeared seizure attacks.

With these results, certain studies indicated that this type of feeding generated molecules called ketones, which were the reason for the success in reducing epileptic seizures; on the other hand, other studies showed that the shortage of glucose is the reason why these seizures were lightened.

Since this diet is low in carbohydrates and abundant in fats, it allows our body to produce molecules (which we could consider a type of fuel) called "ketones." The ketone would be like a kind of alternative fuel, which our body uses when we have glucose (sugar) deficiency in the blood.

This molecule is produced by the liver by decreasing the intake of carbohydrates and proteins, as they become sugar when absorbed into our bloodstream. As we saw before, ketone becomes a kind of fuel for our body in general, but especially produces a large amount of fuel for our brain. As we know, the brain is considered a kind of computer in our body, this is responsible for processing all kinds of information such as movements, gestures, every word we say or think in our day to day, which is why this organ needs more energy consumption, which in this case would be ketone or glucose.

When we apply the ketogenic diet, our body changes the way we supply that "fuel" to work mainly with the fat we produce. This is burned constantly 24 hours a day, every day of the week. This happens when our insulin levels drop because our body is given access to that fat stored in the body to be burned.

The ketogenic diet is ideal if you need to lose weight as it provides a lot of benefits such as improved concentration, improved energy supply, and something very obvious, feeling more satisfied with each meal.

When we eat this type of diet, our body enters a metabolic state called ketosis, which is nothing more than a natural state in which our body feeds itself entirely on fat.

There are some restrictions on this type of diet. Definitively we can say that the ketogenic diet possesses a great number of benefits. However, this also possesses a certain quantity of "negative" effects, which indicate that their practice could come to be considered dangerous for some people since it influences as much in physical health as their mental health.

To correctly follow the ketogenic diet we must take into account that we will make certain changes in our lifestyle, and therefore we must be prepared physically and mentally for it, this is why it is not recommended to start with this type of food to those people who still consider the excessive consumption of carbohydrates as a fundamental part of their diet, people seeking a temporary solution to lose weight, people who do not maintain a constant routine (as we saw earlier when practicing this diet, our body enters a state of ketosis, and our body needs to be able to adapt to the changes).

In particular, this type of diet is not recommended to all those people who are taking medication or have a special health condition, pregnant women or mothers who are breastfeeding.

WHO SHOULD FOLLOW THIS DIET?

This diet is mostly recommended for all epileptic patients, although most young people find it difficult to follow this type of diet, due to the fact that it requires strict compliance with the way of eating.

Among the possible side effects of this diet are growth retardation (when this diet is applied to children), kidney problems, weight loss, bone weakness, etc.

When a person with an epileptic condition is willing to follow this diet, he or she must spend a few days in the hospital in order to monitor the possible effects to which his or her body may react. Once this has happened, you should have constant control with a nutritionist who can guide the patient on how to serve their portions of food.

PEOPLE WITH TYPE 1 DIABETES

We know that this type 1 diabetes is an autoimmune disease, where the immune system attacks the pancreas, destroying the cells that detect sugar in the blood and are responsible for creating insulin; when this happens, the body is unable to absorb glucose, and the accumulated sugar could increase in a very dangerous way.

Therefore, patients with type 1 diabetes must maintain constant monitoring of their blood sugar levels; in addition, they must inject certain amounts of insulin to regulate this. This disease is very common in adults over 30 years old, although there are cases of people whose disease was detected in childhood.

People who suffer from this can present complications in their organism, such as hypertension, eye damage, damage to the nervous system, damage to the renal system, and can even develop heart disease. It is for this reason that the ketogenic diet can greatly influence its improvement since by lowering blood sugar, the need for insulin would be reduced by up to 70%; clearly, this must always be with absolutely strict obedience to the ketogenic diet.

It is very important to stick to this diet because if you fail or cheat with some food, you could put your body in a dangerous and deadly state known as ketoacidosis; this happens when ketone molecules accumulate in the blood, reacting in an aggressive way and making this blood become acidic.

PEOPLE WITH TYPE 2 DIABETES

This type of diabetes is the result of a bad nutritional lifestyle in which sugar levels are elevated to very high levels, thus creating insulin resistance, this is nothing more than an inability on the part of the body to make use of the hormone that produces insulin.

It could be very contradictory to apply the ketogenic diet to type 2 diabetic patients, as most of these are patients with obesity, and adding a diet high in fat would be somewhat confusing. But this could be seen as a misunderstanding in the information of carbohydrates and calories as they are not all the same.

Calories, unlike carbohydrates, are capable of reducing appetite, causing a type 2 diabetic to reduce his or her calorie intake. Additionally, it also decreases the production of ghrelin; this is informally known as the hormone that produces appetite, and it also increases the production of amylin and leptin; informally known as the hormones that make us feel satisfied as a result of ketosis.

Type 2 diabetes patients are also very susceptible to ketoacidosis, so it is very important that they are in constant medical checkups and maintain a balanced diet provided by a nutritionist.

CHAPTER 2: KETO MYTHS

Because this type of diet may look a little strict or a lot, depending on your point of view, many myths arise about the keto diet. Like the following:

- When you enter ketosis, your body goes towards ketoacidosis: What does this mean? For as you already know, ketosis means that blood sugar levels are low, so the body goes into ketosis, turning fat into energy; if that's the case, you can start losing fat and so on, but now ketoacidosis is something absolutely different, because this is a medical condition, which is extremely serious, because it is produced by low levels of insulin, and very, very high levels of ketones, which could become fatal, we can say that this condition is found in some diabetic patients. Seeing both concepts, we can observe that they are diametrically different things, since one is a healthy condition of the body, which allows the burning of fats in a natural way, and the other is a clinical condition of patients with diabetes.
- The keto diet is based only on the elimination of carbohydrates: This is completely false, since the basis of the keto diet is not only that but is also based on a very high consumption of fats, in addition, it does not seek to eliminate by complete carbohydrates, but requires an efficient consumption of them, the minimum really, but does not prohibit the consumption of them, since it is based on a set of conditions that must be met to get to ketosis, which involves obtaining energy through fat and not sugars that provide us with carbohydrates.
- Muscle is lost while doing the ketogenic diet: This is false, because the keto, is extremely used for athletes, but this myth arises from a confusion, because there is a process in the body, which converts protein into glucose, and as you know, our body is not able to break down fat into glucose. For this reason people think that muscle would be lost, but they can not be further from reality, since almost nothing is converted into glucose, for this reason, it is understood that you get to the false conclusion that you lose muscle, but for the muscles to be maintained, or grow, it is something absolutely amazing, because to get started, the muscles necessarily use glucose, therefore, there are processes in our body that are dependent on glucose, but there are others that are not, and the same tasks that some organs can perform with glucose, they can perform with ketones, one of these organs capable of doing this is the brain, the amazing process that the human body is the following, the little glucose that the body generates goes to the brain, but in this case, the brain depends on ketones, and a certain amount of them will go to the brain, and the glucose that was intended for that organ, will go to the muscles, so as to maintain muscle mass or increase the size of them.

- All people need the same amounts of carbohydrates: This is totally false since not everyone has the same needs because they depend on the individual health conditions of each person. Therefore, it is likely that some people will not be able to make a strict ketogenic diet right away, as they may be affected by such a drastic change in their dietary intake, this may also depend on their daily physical activity.
- The ketogenic diet limits the consumption of certain foods: This is absolutely true, as many of the foods it restricts are cereals, sweets, sugary drinks, processed foods and lots of fruits, as most of its composition is based on carbohydrates, thus becoming, into fructose in the body and making the process of ketosis more difficult, and that energy would not be produced thanks to fats and ketones, but to sugars in our body.
- The ketogenic diet slows down your metabolism: This is because when people hear the word diet, comes to mind the slowing of the metabolism, and this is because, in the vast majority of diets, a large decrease in calorie consumption, in the long run, will generate a slowing of the metabolism of people who make such diets. In order to avoid this and make use of ketosis, it is good that one day, we proceed to eat carbohydrates, of course not in a big excess, but you will skip the diet, so to speak. After that, you can resume ketosis, because there will come a time when you can reach the state of ketosis very quickly. But it is that really, this diet has something very particular, since this allows to maintain the same metabolism or could even increase it, since it makes a high consumption of calories, and allows you to lose weight, thus achieving to be a diet that carries out something totally different to the other diets, because the common ones are characterized by a low caloric consumption and these are able to slow down the metabolism. Although we already mentioned that the ketogenic diet does not slow down the metabolism, it is not a bad practice, as previously said, to consume sometimes a greater amount of carbohydrates.
- Eating so many fats is harmful to health: This is a myth, since there are good fats and bad fats, which are harmful are those found in frying oils, butter and trans fats, but there are also good fats, those found in food without the need to go through chemical processes, such as avocados, coconut oil, among others, as there are many people who believe they have to eat fried foods, butter, hamburgers, pizzas, because the ketogenic diet is based on the consumption of fats, but on the good consumption of them. Good fats are vital to the body for various reasons, among which are found to be responsible for the constitution of cell membranes, transport fat-soluble vitamins, and as if this were not enough, also provides energy to the body. Therefore, we can say that the human body needs fats for its proper functioning, but in a good proportion.
- Ketogenic diets are high in protein: This is false for several reasons, the first is that a high intake of protein is going to become fructose or sugar in our blood so to speak,

which causes it to leave the state of ketosis, therefore, affects the purpose of the diet, which is to get to be at that level to burn fat, another point that affects the high intake of protein, is that the decomposition of amino acids that are obtained in proteins, produce an increase in the number of ketones found in our body, but although this sounds attractive for the purposes of the keto diet, the same is hazardous to health, since a disproportionate amount of ketones in our body more than a benefit can become a risk.

- The ketogenic diet involves not eating for long periods of time: This is false, since this type of diet never requires long periods of time without eating, but rather a low-carbohydrate diet, which is the basis of the keto diet, but although there is no restriction when consuming food, it is also true that fasting is very useful and beneficial to lose weight, but the fundamental principle of keto, is to make a complete food plan, which allows people to nourish themselves and feel satiated when eating, consuming quality fat, thus producing high levels of energy that do not depend on the fructose generated by carbohydrates, but fat, thanks to ketones
- The ketogenic diet does not allow to consume sweets or desserts: This is false, since the keto, is based on not consuming carbohydrates or processed foods such as sugars, but there are desserts that do not have anything of that in their preparation, such as those based on nuts, Greek yogurt, chocolate, in addition, that these are sweetened with natural sweeteners such as stevia, because as you know, it does not have fructose. Therefore, we can get sweets such as cheesecakes, brownies, or even biscuits, and there is no need for any of the traditional ingredients that would take us out of the state of ketosis. These recipes will be explained later, as the book progresses.

These are some of the myths that we can get with the ketogenic diet, as you can see, there are still people who do not believe in it by this type of myth, it will only depend on you whether to believe in the keto or not.

CHAPTER 3: BENEFITS OF USING KETO

When we talk about ketogenic feeding we can think that the only benefit or the one that stands out, at first sight, is the considerable weight loss, which is in fact achieved quickly, but not only is the weight loss the benefit that is achieved with this diet, as we have commented previously, in its beginnings this diet was applied in adults and children who suffered from epileptic seizures.

Improvements have also been observed in people suffering from convulsions and problems in their cognitive functions.

It has also been noted that in people who have certain brain conditions, the keto diet has some curative properties when done, such as neurodegenerative diseases, epilepsy. In addition to being able to raise endorphin levels, thus raising moods, as well as improvements in concentration, raises melatonin levels, helping to better sleep and regulate our circadian cycle.

In addition, this diet considerably lowers blood sugar levels, which is why it is widely recommended for diabetics. This is mainly due to the fact that by decreasing carbohydrate consumption, we are going to decrease blood sugar levels. When we eat carbohydrates, these foods are digested and transformed into glucose in the blood, in that sense starts to act insulin which is the hormone that is responsible for sending all that glucose to cells to consume it or in its absence and that is actually what always happens, to be stored. There are cases in which the cells stop responding to insulin, and in this way, the control of glucose in the blood is lost, and this is when we have a serious problem because we would be talking about suffering from type 2 diabetes. But in patients who have been treated with this ketogenic diet and exercise, considerable improvements have been found. In fact, many of the people have considerably decreased the consumption of their medications since applying it.

Cardiovascular improvements are also obtained, thus improving all the indicators that determine the risk of suffering cardiovascular diseases, it has been shown in various studies that although this diet increases fat consumption, cholesterol levels improve, this means that there is a higher percentage of good cholesterol HDL and LDL-C, there is also a large decrease in triglyceride levels and improvements in blood pressure of people who practice it. Against all odds when some critics thought that this type of food could alter cholesterol levels and triglycerides, as it has been determined that the opposite happens.

Taking the body to the state of ketosis one of the most noticeable changes is the decrease in body fat and less visceral fat, the subcutaneous fat is the fat that we can feel or in its defect pinch and that we can get in our arms, legs, belly and other places. While visceral fat is that it accumulates around the organs and that could, in some cases, cause us or increase health risks. With this feeding method, we are able to reduce these two types of fat. Especially there is a considerable decrease in fat in the abdominal cavity.

Ketogenic diets have been used for many years to treat epilepsy problems, but this type of diet is also being studied for diseases such as Alzheimer's, Parkinson's, and this is because ketogenic bodies have neuroprotective effects.

And is that one of the benefits of the keto diet, it has the possibility to feed and heal the brain, this diet is the main source of energy of the brain.

The digestive system is considered as the second brain we have, the intestine has a structure like a mesh, and this mesh is pierced or perforated by anti-nutrients and gluten, which is what is known in medicine as a permeable intestine, this pathology achieves an inflammatory process in the body that is able to improve with the keto, this diet is able to help regulate the digestive system.

Dopamine is a molecule produced in a natural way by our organism, within its functions we have the pleasure, learning, decision making, coordination of movements, motivation, and when we are in the presence of dopamine the reward systems of our brain are going to activate and in this way respond the stimulus that has a positive charge in each one of us. Dopamine helps in the process of remembering some information. Now the low levels of dopamine are directly related to states of depression, attention deficit disorders, hyperactivity, Parkinson's, hyperthyroidism. But the good news is that the keto diet increases dopamine levels, so it's advisable to eat this way.

When we reach the level of ketosis, there are many advantages and benefits that we acquire with this. There is a decrease in inflammation at a general level in the body, decreases oxidative stress, being these neuroprotective, antitumor. It increases our immune system, so we can conclude that another benefit is to improve autoimmune diseases.

With all that we have mentioned previously we cannot consider the ketogenic diet only to lose weight, we already know that it is a diet that metabolizes fat in an effective and efficient way, if we have an excess of fat our body will use it, otherwise it will use the fat you eat as a fuel and when it needs more fuel will let you know through hunger.

Reaching these ketogenic levels enhances the physical and mental performance of each one of those who practice it, and this is because, in ketosis, blood glucose levels are always stable, so we will not suffer from symptoms of hypoglycemia. We become healthier, and in addition, we do not have any secondary effect, the key is not to fail, is to achieve in principle to detoxify our body of all the antinutrients that are hosted in the body, once achieved this step we will see how easy it is to implement this food plan.

Migraines are classified as a neurological disorder, the lack of energy in neurons is one of the causes of these migraines, it is well known that there are many treatments that have been tried for migraines, but we have good news, ketosis can eliminate this disorder, hypoglycemia is associated with headache, when we are on a normal diet, glucose is the sole fuel for the brain, so the energy we need for neurons is not enough, but this does not happen with ketones, as an alternative fuel. Since ketones are then the most effective fuel for the brain, the heart, and also the intestine, they preserve and promote the creation of muscle mass, promote the generation of new mitochondria, and finally increases longevity in each of the people who practice it.

The ketogenic diet activates the necessary genes to be able to use fat as the main fuel, and sugar as a secondary fuel, so we can say that we are going to have two fuel tanks, one coming from fats where millions of kcal can be stored, and another tank of sugar or glycogen and which is also very limited since it has approximately 2000 kcal. When we use the sugar tank we spend it quickly so we will need to refill this tank and get again the fuel we need, but if on the contrary, we use fat fuel with the keto diet, we will have an inexhaustible tank of fuel and available at any time, could there be a better benefit of it?. The keto diet is a wonderful tool to improve our health.

CHAPTER 4: KETOSIS AND MENTAL HEALTH

To begin this section, the first thing we need to know or define is, what is health? And what is a better definition than what the world health organization can offer us? It says that literally "Health is a state of complete physical, mental and social well-being, and not only the absence of disease or illness", therefore, we can say that health is not only the lack of physical illnesses, but that one must also be mentally and psychologically balanced, in addition to being socially good with others, since many studies have shown that a person who is not psychologically well will not have physical health either. Moreover, cancer patients often make psychological therapies so that they can recover faster since emotionally stable patients have a higher percentage of recovery.

Therefore, we recommend that you first try to be mentally stable because no matter how much ketogenic diet you do, you will not be able to have a complete integral health, therefore it is always good to have the three stable states of health, both physical, emotional and social.

After having mentioned the importance of the integral health, we can explain the importance of the ketogenic diet to be able to improve our physical health, since this not only helps us to reduce, since many times, this is the end that is sought to the diets, but the same one has a number of utilities in the scope of the health as you will be able to see next.

Ketosis and Cancer: The keto diet is very useful for cancer patients, because a large part of cancer cells feed on glucose cells and as you should already know that glucose in our body is produced thanks to carbohydrate intake, therefore by drastically lowering their consumption, fewer glucose cells will be created, and the cancer cells will not be able to feed, or not most of them, since almost none of these cells can feed on ketones, so we can stop or slow down the growth rate of the cancer.

Ketosis and diabetes: As you should know, diabetes is a disease that occurs when there is an excessive concentration of glucose in the blood, either because the pancreas does not make enough insulin, and this generates that glucose is not transformed into energy efficiently. Therefore, after knowing this, we can make use of the keto diet, and thus achieve control of glucose in our blood, because we will generate more ketones in our body, and these will do the work of glucose in our body, generating energy through them, thus achieving a better quality of life for patients.

But now, going to the point, ketosis has a great impact on our brain health since first, much of the vital processes for our body is done by the brain with the help of ketosis, but these functions can also be used with the help of ketones. Therefore, we can say that the brain can use the cells that are produced when practicing the ketogenic diet to perform their vital functions.

One of the first benefits we can see from the ketogenic diet is that it improves the condition of patients suffering from epilepsy, which is a brain disorder that occurs when there is electrical overactivity in some specific areas of the brain, people who suffer from this, may suffer convulsions or unwanted movements, when these seizures occur are called epileptic seizures. But then, for a treatment, or help that can be done to patients suffering from epilepsy, is the use of the ketogenic diet, since the diet is able to reduce to a very high degree the frequency of seizures that can occur to patients suffering from epilepsy, of course this does not mean that patients should stop taking their pills to control the disease, but the keto diet could be a great help in reducing the frequency of seizures, because as you know, the ketogenic diet makes a high increase in the level of ketones in the blood, thus making a better control of seizures.

Most of the time this diet is prescribed, it is scoped for children, and the statistical results of patients with epilepsy, we can find that there are cases that range between 10% and 15% who do not suffer from seizures again, there are also other cases in which more than 50% of patients who are instructed to follow the diet, the frequency in which seizures occur is reduced to at least half the time. How does the ketogenic diet help patients with seizures? Well, since we have a high level of ketosis, it allows us to alter the genes that are related to the brain's energetic metabolism, since the brain will take ketones as its main source of nutrition, instead of glucose, which implies that neuronal functions will be controlled, which are those that are affected at the time of the seizures. Also to verify the result of the keto diet in our brain, regarding that disease, we can observe that there was a substantial increase in the energy reserves of the neurons of the hippocampus, increasing the number of mitochondria, therefore, increasing the concentration of mitochondria in the hippocampus, meaning that the density of mitochondria in the hippocampus increased a lot, this means that energy production in the hippocampus is improved, which may mean that better neuronal stability will be obtained.

On the other hand there are other brain diseases that can be improved through the practice of the ketogenic diet, such as Alzheimer, which is a brain disease, better said is a progressive cognitive disorder that will degenerate brain cells, which leads to problems of memory, thinking, and behavior, such disease is gradually worsening, leading to the death of people suffering from that disease. There is no way to end the disease, there are only treatments to slow its degenerative process, but there is no way to eliminate it. But in order for these patients to achieve a better quality of life, the ketogenic diet can be recommended, since the ketones in the brain could reactivate some neurons, thus repairing part of the brain damage caused by Alzheimer's, since thanks to the help of ketones, we can try to prolong the life of these neurons, also taking care of our dendrites and axons, thus achieving, or better said, trying to achieve better connections in the brain to try to make synapses. This being the main damage of Alzheimer's disease, as it does not allow a good synapse in the brain, thus placing increasingly difficult barriers in patients to use their brain, either to remember things or do daily activities. Although it cannot be said that there is irrefutable evidence that the ketogenic diet can stop Alzheimer's or put an end to it, what we can say is that they have carried out a series of experiments on animals, which already have brain degeneration, something very similar to those suffered by these types of patients, and it can be said that the animals that were on a ketogenic diet, could perform the tasks in a better way to the animals that were not on it; on the other hand, studies were made on mice in their juvenile stage, which had brain lesions, and it could be observed that those to whom the ketogenic diet was applied, the brain was protected from damage, but not only that, there were cases in which it was possible to regenerate brain damage. Therefore, we can say that the ketogenic diet could be hopeful for those patients suffering from Alzheimer's disease.

These are some of the diseases with which the ketogenic diet can help us, but there are also others that would be just as useful to have a better quality of life, to mention some other brain disease that this diet could help brain cancer could be one of them, by this we do not mean that the diseases are eliminated only by making the diet, because it is not magic either, but we can say that it could improve the quality of life of the patient, and it is also very good for the patient to be in better condition to take the treatment with his doctor of confidence.

CHAPTER 5: KETOGENIC NUTRITION

When starting a ketogenic diet, we must take into account very important factors such as our dietary habits; the amount of food we eat each day with its consistency (this includes heavy or light meals).

In addition, we must take into account important factors of our body, such as our body weight and height, consider if we are consuming any pharmacological treatment, perform previous blood tests to discard any weakness that may occur in our body.

The ketogenic diet has an innumerable variety of benefits, we have already seen how it can improve brain functions, helps hormonal regulation in women, has been used for patients suffering from epileptic seizures, and so an endless list of benefits that has managed to place this diet as one of the most requested and as one of the most researched.

But it has also arisen the need to know if this method of feeding possesses nutrients of high value for our organism, and is that although the main restriction of the keto diet is the elimination of the carbohydrates and of the refined sugars and flours, the foods that are allowed are of high nutritional content.

If we learn to know our body and the nutritional contents of food, we can make a significant change in our lives. One of the food groups that is consumed most in this diet is vegetables. It is recommended to consume many green foods, such as spinach, celery, or celery, Spain, parsley, all with high nutritional properties and large amounts of magnesium.

Another of the foods that are used in this plan is the consumption of meat, chicken, pork or fish, although in other diets this type of food is restricted, this is a diet that prioritizes the consumption of natural and healthy fats, without affecting cholesterol levels or triglyceride levels, whitefish are lean options that are both reduced calories, fish is a high-quality protein and a wonderful source of omega 3, which provides innumerable benefits for the health of our body, the main idea of ketogenic food is to reduce as much as possible the consumption of carbohydrates to be able to produce ketone bodies or ketosis.

Olive oil is a key element and nutritious, is an excellent source of quality fat for the body, olive oil has antioxidant and anti-inflammatory properties. It is also a high-quality oil, but it is always advisable to use it in a moderate way and avoid fried foods when preparing meals.

The avocado is a fruit widely used in this diet, is a vegetable protein that provides antioxidant benefits as well as vitamins and minerals, the avocado is rich in potassium, in addition to having fatty acids that are very beneficial for cardiovascular health, have a large amount of fiber, help lower cholesterol levels and triglycerides. It is a food that you can use to prepare breakfast, lunch, or dinner, and as you can see, the food is also focused on improving your health.

The egg is also an allowed food and provides us fat and protein, vitamin B1, A, D, B2, and niacin, with which we can make a lot of dishes, and complements for other meals.

Nuts and seeds are also recommended in this diet, rich in fiber and natural fats, omega3, antioxidants, in addition to seeds and nuts can make a large number of dishes, whether keto bread, tortillas, butter, and even chocolate creams, because as you acquire more knowledge on the subject and the properties of the food you are consuming, you can be able to prepare dishes or highly nutritious menus and with the goal of finally reaching nutritional ketosis.

Fresh cheeses are rich in protein with a low amount of saturated fat and sodium, are a rich source of calcium, vitamin A and D. There are also vegan cheeses that, in addition to being very rich, there is a wide variety of them.

in the ketogenic diet there are different types within it, there is the classic ketogenic diet rich in fat, where about 90% of the diet consumed is fat, this diet is adjusted to the energy amounts of each individual, in general, it is managed in the following way: for every 3 or 4 grams of fat consumed, a gram of protein is offered together. however, this is not always the case, depending on the needs of each person, the diet will be adjusted depending on its ketogenic capacity.

There is also the ketogenic diet with medium-chain triglycerides MCT diet proposed in 1971 by Huttenlocher. In this diet, the type of fat is consumed as MCT oil, and it is that MCT lipids are metabolized faster than long-chain triglycerides LCT, and thus allow ketosis more quickly.

WHAT STEPS SHOULD BE FOLLOWED FOR THE PROPER FUNCTION OF THIS DIET?

As the ketogenic diet is a complex level diet, it is very important that each step is strictly followed without any mistakes.

It does not matter if we make this diet by our own decision or to improve our health and physical condition or if we suffer from some type of disease (such as epilepsy, diabetes among others) which would benefit us in health, it is very important to go to a nutritionist to give us the necessary guidance not to harm our health and to inform us correctly how to follow the ketogenic diet.

In the case of children, it is very important that they comply with all the rules of the balanced diet without any failure; since, as they are in a growth stage, these changes will mark a great change in their organism and cognitive development. As we already know, each diet is personal, and for this reason, not all diets are appropriate for all children (regardless of whether they are the same age, weight or size).

Nutritionists usually mainly evaluate the number of nutrients consumed in the first three days of starting this new style of nutrition in order to observe in detail how our body reacts to the changes and even in some cases, supervises a disease.

TYPES OF KETOGENIC DIET

There are different types of cytogenetic diet, and that is why we must be very attentive to which is the most appropriate according to our physical and mental condition.

CYCLIC CYTOGENETIC DIET

This type of diet is one in which, as its name says, a cycle is going to be followed in which a plan of certain periods for consuming carbohydrates is included, for example: 6 days of strict compliance with the ketogenic diet and one day of carbohydrates.

STANDARD KETOGENIC DIET

This is the type of diet where your low-carbohydrate meal plan moderates carbohydrate intake and most foods will be fat-based. This will normally range from 75% to 80% fat, 15% to 20% protein and only 5% or less carbohydrate intake.

HIGH PROTEIN KETOGENIC DIET

This type of diet is one in which food distribution is as follows: 60% fat, 5% carbohydrate, and 35% protein. In other words, this diet will be performing the functions of the standard cytogenetic diet but will add more protein than usual.

It is important to note that these percentages may vary according to the needs of our body and condition.

ADAPTED CYTOGENETIC DIET

This is the type of diet in which we are allowed to consume carbohydrates on the days we exercise.

Mostly, cyclic or adapted diets are used for more professional purposes by health experts, athletes or bodybuilders as they have a deeper knowledge of their body and are able to handle any type of situation with their body.

CHAPTER 6: INTERMITTENT FASTING

Increasingly more people are interested in practicing intermittent fasting, as every day are more known the broad benefits that can be achieved by our body to apply it. Today, the word "intermittent fasting" has practically become a worldwide trend, particularly in the field of fitness and methods to lose weight more quickly and without rebound effect, which is what mainly concerns people who make different diets.

Intermittent fasting is a physiological mechanism that has been practiced since our ancestors, fasting is absolutely beneficial to health, and is something that has been practiced throughout history.

But which are the results that we can obtain when applying the intermittent fast, that encourages us to apply it, well, the intermittent fast regulates the glucose in blood, improves the arterial pressure, improves the focus and mental clarity, helps notably in the process of detoxification, increases considerably the levels of energy of our body, increases the productivity of different hormones in our organism, like the growth hormone, reduces the rate of aging, prevents the cancer, cellular regeneration, among many of the other benefits.

Intermittent fasting is very important and consists of not eating food for an estimated time. Fasting daily between 16-22 hours is a health tool that decreases the risk of disease.

When we do the intermittent fasting insulin levels go down when these levels go down, the body draws energy from the liver and fats, and when we fast continuously our body will achieve a good balance and begins the keto-adaptation. Intermittent fasting works because when we lower insulin levels, the body begins to burn fat.

The best way to go with intermittent fasting is with the ketogenic diet, exercise. Intermittent fasting allows the hormones to do their job correctly, during this period of time that we do not ingest any food there is no insulin, and in its absence, counter-regulating hormones such as growth hormone, glucagon, adrenaline, etc., can initiate pathways for cell repair and thus clean our body of metabolic waste, helping the growth of muscle mass, to access our body fat that begins to be intelligently used by our body as energy, begins the production of ketones in the liver and increases basal caloric expenditure.

When we fast intermittently, increases the production of growth hormones (GH), as mentioned above, but what does this hormone do in our body? does three fundamental things: it favors lipolysis, increasing the oxidation of fats, thus helping the production of ketones, also helps maintain muscle mass inhibiting muscle degradation to make glucose, and finally prevents us from presenting symptoms of hypoglycemia.

We have to understand that when we eat and when we suppress ourselves from food we generate hormones that have different mechanisms of action, for example, when we practice fasting, meaning that we do not eat for certain periods of time, we generate more growth hormones, adrenaline or glucagon, while when we feed, we generate insulin hormone. At present, people are suffering from hyperinsulinemia and growth hormone deficiency, which leads us to conclude that it is necessary and advisable to apply intermittent fasting accompanied by ketogenic feeding.

There are currently various modalities of intermittent fasting, but we will mention the three most important, remember that it is not a rule to apply and that everyone can apply it according to their own requirements and the recommendations of the specialist. The categories of intermittent fasting that we have summarized among so many types of fasting that there are are are the following:

INTERMITTENT FASTING (IF)

This voluntary fast restricts the intake of solid food for a period of time between 16-48 hours. You can also restrict the consumption of food for a period of time of 6-8 hours.

PERIODIC FASTING (PF)

Buchinger type fast. Büchinger's fasting method consists of a limited intake of fruit juices as well as small amounts of vegetable broth being the nutritional energy consumption of 200 to 400 kcal/day. Exercise is also practiced with this method, mind-body techniques, the application of enemas and the taking of laxative salts.

INTERMEDIATE 24/7 FASTING

This type of intermittent fasting consists of having only 4 hours a day to eat, thus leaving the other 20 hours of fasting; this could be summed up as two meals and even one per day.

This type of fast could offer very promising results because, as we have seen, it is very difficult to be surpassed with food feeding us at most twice a day.

Now, the implementation of any of these types of fasting carries with it a series of results that have been cataloged as beneficial:

On the circadian rhythm, a study with overweight individuals ate for only 10-11 hours a day for 16 weeks and not only they were able to reduce body weight, burn localized fat and manifest to be full of energy, in addition, there were improvements in sleep, and the benefits persisted for one year.

The most common eating pattern in society today is to eat three meals a day plus snacks, in animal and human studies suggest that intermittent fasting, when the fasting period is extended to 16 hours, can improve health indicators and thus counteract disease processes. Changes in fat metabolism occur, and ketones are produced, as well as stimulation of adaptive cellular stress responses that prevent and also repair molecular damage.

Improvements in the antitumor effect have been observed, improving the mechanisms of autophagy, due to these studies Yoshinori Ohsumi has been awarded the Nobel Prize in 2016

Intermittent fasting and fasting itself has the potential to delay aging, and especially brain aging, in animal studies, it has been shown that daily caloric restriction, intermittent fasting, and fasting on alternate days, modifies the sensory pathways of nutrients in the brain, increasing synaptic plasticity, neurogenesis, and neuroprotection.

Recent small trials of intermittent fasting in patients with cancer or multiple sclerosis have generated promising results that provide a strong rationale for moving forward with larger clinical trials.

WHAT IS AUTOPHAGY?

Our organism requires periods of maximum intensity and periods of absolute rest, and we can notice this in the bright light we receive during the day, where many chemical, physiological and biological processes occur in our organism, and later we have a period of rest, when night arrives, where certain processes also occur, the same thing happens with temperature changes and the same thing happens with food, the body needs moments or periods of food nutrition but also needs periods of abstinence and regeneration. When we practice intermittent fasting, for example, we give our body those periods it needs.

When we practice intermittent fasting, something called autophagy occurs, and it can be explained in the following way: in 1974, Christian de Duve discovered the lysosomes, and observed that they had the capacity to recycle cellular scrap, that is, dysfunctional mitochondria, bacteria, and even viruses, and converted them into new functional molecules.

In this way, the cell would be feeding on its own damaged parts to renew itself, and hence the term or expression "autophagy." If we did not live this important process of autophagy in the cells, all that cellular scrap would accumulate in our organism causing finally an endless number of diseases and the accelerated aging of the cellular organism.

When we practice fasting, we activate autophagy, and as a consequence of this activation, all the benefits that were mentioned before are achieved. But autophagy does not occur instantaneously by applying intermittent fasting. Rather it is a process that will occur gradually. It is important to emphasize that it is not necessary to do very prolonged fasting in order to reach autophagy; what is important is to be constant with the implementation of intermittent fasting, for example.

You can start implementing 13-hour fasting in the hours of sleep; you can play with different combinations of intermittent fasting:

Elevated frequency: Periods of 12/12 or 16/8, meaning 12 hours of fasting and 12 hours of food intake within the ketogenic diet, or 16 hours of fasting and 8 hours of food intake within the ketogenic diet. This process can be applied several days a week or every day.

Average frequency: Fasting for 24 hours, this type of fast can be done once a week, it should be noted that this kind of practice is recommended to be performed under medical supervision and with prior preparation of our body, it is not recommended under any circumstances to practice without prior information.

Low frequency: fasting or restricting the consumption of solid food for 2-3 days and generally practiced once a month; likewise, this type of practice should be performed under medical supervision.

During fasting, you can consume water, apple vinegar, coffee, water with lemon, tea, but the fat, coconut oil, and green juices do come out of fasting, as carbohydrates and fat stimulate insulin.

How can we break these hours of fasting? Once we spend hours without eating solid food. Autophagy is inhibited by elevations of insulin or the presence of amino acids, but it is very difficult to determine. During fasting is advisable to consume water to which you can add lemon or orange juice, probiotic drinks, bone broth that provides nutrition with the intake of few calories. These are some of the combinations of foods that we recommend to break the fast, since when so many hours go by without ingesting solid foods it is not recommended that when finishing it, one begins ingesting great amounts of food but rather to begin with a tea, a broth of bones, water, and gradually starts ingesting foods within the ketogenic diet.

Fasting is contraindicated for pregnant women, children, anyone who has hormonal alterations, are some of the contraindications that we must take into account before applying the fast, which is why we insist on the fact that before fasting should be consulted with experts because each case is individual.

CHAPTER 7: BENEFITS OF FASTING

THE ADVANTAGES OF FASTING

One of the most obvious advantages of fasting is weight loss. In ancient times it was called detoxification of the body to all periods of fasting in which the idea was to limit the intake of food for a certain number of hours in order to purify the digestive system. It was believed that if you lasted a while detoxifying, our body will remove all those toxins from it and make us look younger. In a way was right because living a healthy lifestyle, our skin is the first to reflect it.

The correct follow-up of this routine of feeding can offer us a number of benefits to health and even to our physical performance in the day to day. As has been mentioned, the results of these benefits will be those that depend on our willingness to improve eating habits.

This is why when we make a food protocol such as intermittent fasting, we must do it in a proper way because it is useless to fast based on a diet of pre-cooked food, junk, fried and canned or any other food of non-natural origin, since it is going to be the same as continuing to consume these foods in our day to day, every day.

Among the advantages of intermittent fasting that benefits our organism is the following:

- It improves the sensitivity of insulin and glucose as an energy substrate:

As mentioned above, insulin is that hormone produced by the pancreas, which is responsible for capturing glucose as a result of carbohydrate intake (which are stored in the blood to be subsequently released and transported to the point where they will be used to balance glucose levels).

When this hormone becomes so sensitive to our body, there is a higher burning of fat accumulated in our body as a result of the decrease in glycogen within our body in the period of fasting (especially when doing some physical activity). It is for this reason that our body is able to assimilate in a more effective way the glucose that we provide at-home food.

- It helps to lose fat, improve cholesterol, and reduce triglycerides.

As we have mentioned before, one of the main reasons why many people come to this diet looking for a way to burn fat and also improve cholesterol and reduce triglycerides.

Many studies state that physical activity and intermittent fasting can achieve greater fat loss, in turn improving the body system.

- Increases SIRT3, the protein of youth, and reduces mortality.

When our body is in a state of fasting, our body performs a series of processes that favor the growth hormone and youth protein. This hormone makes it difficult for our body to consume glucose, and that is why it is forced to resort to the reserve of accumulated fat in order to obtain energy.

- It helps to reduce the growth of cancer cells.

Fasting is considered a way to reduce the possibility of cancer because when glucose is absent, all those healthy cells automatically begin to burn fat, thus leaving the cancer cells without energy and oxidized to kill them completely.

It also reduces the levels of IGF-1, a hormone linked to insulin, which is considered an engine of cell proliferation considered necessary at the time of physical activity. However, its level can be dangerous when a person has already developed cancer.

- It helps to reduce mortality due to obesity problems.

It has been proven that intermittent fasting can be a good method of disease prevention (which is preventive in the long term). Although it is known that suffering from obesity increases the scope to all types of diseases (heart, glycaemic and many others) which can be deadly, the correct observance of a fast can reduce considerably (or in its entirety) the concentrations of triacylglycerol, the increase in cholesterol and glucose level and can even reduce the possibility of developing diseases such as Alzheimer's disease.

In addition, among the advantages that favor us, the following factors are noteworthy:

- Reduces inflammation.
- It helps us to improve our capacity for self-control in the face of anxiety and lack of food control.
- It has positive effects on the neuronal system.
- It favors autophagy; the organism activates internal recycling mechanisms.

Many investigations have shown that most people prefer to follow an intermittent fasting regime in their long-term eating habits to follow a diet that generates anxiety in terms of food restriction.

These investigations also show that reducing only the intake of calories in their daily diet facilitates much more in the preparation of their food; there have been cases of people who used to consume infinite calories and with only reducing a few have managed to improve their habits without feeling the absence of their dietary change and even achieving a massive loss of weight or excessive fat.

How Does Intermittent Fasting Affect Our Body?

The intermittent fast, in addition to restricting the intake of calories, benefits the hormones of the body to resort to the accumulated fat. In addition, fasting greatly favors the regeneration of those damaged cells of our body.

As for the sensitivity of insulin, it is able to help all (or most) people who suffer from problems of overweight to burn fat more quickly and effectively. Also, while burning fat, at the same time, is generating muscle and that is why these types of diet are more used by bodybuilders and athletes.

Is Intermittent Fasting Recommended for Anyone Who Practices Physical Activity?

As we have been talking about, there is no specific training routine or diet because each person's body assimilates things differently. What we must take into account is that when doing a very intense training (whether cycling, swimming, or running in a marathon) is necessary to consume something that gives us a good performance and, in this case, a fast would not be ideal for these types of situation.

The same could be applied to people who do not perform physical activities of high performance but mild physical activities, but who perform it in high weather conditions of temperature and humidity, as the body will need the consumption of more energy to adapt to the situation in which it is and will not have sufficient nutrients.

It is for this reason that at the moment of carrying out an intermittent fast, it is necessary to take into account the level of demand, conditions to which we are exposed, and duration during our training. In addition, we must always take into account the time that has elapsed since the last meal until the start of training, making sure that we have digested our food correctly.

Surely we have heard that a training in fast is usually much more recommended and we will think that this is a contradiction, a training in fast is always good for the health of the person as long as the duration of this is equal or less than an hour, with a low intensity (or moderately high). In this way, the body adapts slowly to work in low glycogen conditions.

Fasting when exercising is not recommended for all those who have suffered from any type of eating disorder (such as anorexia or bulimia), people with diabetes or hypoglycemia as it can be harmful to your body.

It is very common to think that this method of intermittent fasting is something new that has been used in recent years, while it is true that it has been a method that has gained popularity in recent years, in fact, this method of feeding comes from primitive times because they had no option to access food and had to go out in search of them.

In the same way, it will always be advisable for each person to evaluate what method can result from this protocol, and in this way, observe how it influences their daily workday or exercise. In this way, you are checking what your body needs and if it is able to handle it.

CHAPTER 8: FASTING FOR WEIGHT LOSS

We already have previous knowledge of what fasting is all about. We know what it means to abstain from eating, drinking or both, for a period of time chosen by the fasting practitioner.

Fasting is a process that has been practiced for many years, from our ancestors and in different cultures, in fact, there are populations that practice fasting and are long-lasting populations, practicing fasting, exercise, and good food. But fasting today is also widely used to lose weight. However, more than a tool to lose weight, it is a lifestyle to improve health, as we have seen in previous cases.

To apply the fast in our organism to lose weight helps to eliminate the accumulated fat of the body and to lose weight, in the same way it helps to take advantage of the energy that is used for the digestion in other processes of the organism, to be able this way to give a rest to some of our organs. The fasting serves to cleanse and detoxify the body. It is always advisable to seek help from specialists before applying fasting because, when applied incorrectly can also have harmful consequences on our body, so it is important not only to investigate but to know our body and be guided by a specialist at the beginning of this very beneficial process.

In order to lose weight, several types of fasting have been implemented:

There are fasts that are applied for a long period, and this fast can last several weeks or even months, depending on the desired results and the physiological conditions of each organism. In this stage, all carbohydrates and calories are eliminated and what is mainly consumed is only liquid. The main objective of this fast is to quickly reach the levels of ketosis in our body. But we must compensate for this lack of food with supplements, minerals guided by specialists, depending exclusively on the conditions and particular requirements of each person.

Juice fasting is a type of fasting in which the main food are fruit juices. There are several fasting protocols like this one that are applied for specific diseases including cancer, a well-known, and applied therapy for healing and detoxification is the "Gerson therapy." In this type of fast, all the necessary nutrients must be incorporated for our bodies. At the same time, it helps the body to improve digestion, and this is achieved in this case by not consuming any solid food.

Alternate fasting is very often used by experts for weight loss and fat burning, in this case, you can get to have a full day without eating food and alternate with normal days where food is consumed in a restricted or controlled way following the ketogenic diet naturally. It is fast, and just like those mentioned above, it must be prescribed by experts. We must have the knowledge not only to follow and stick to them but to get the expected results because if not applied correctly, it can also bring consequences to our health.

Periodic fasting, which differs from intermittent fasting in that this type of fasting is applied for a certain time, but there are more days of normal feeding or where solid foods are allowed, in this case, the fasting can be done on a specific day, could be a specific day a week, for example, and the rest of the week the person has permission to consume the foods permitted within the ketogenic diet.

Intermittent fasting is currently the best known and applied by all or most people who apply the ketogenic diet in which they are going to consume food for a specific period of time, and then spend another period without food or consuming liquids that do not break with the fasting applied, for example, you can fast for 16 hours, managing to stop eating food during that period and after it consuming food within the ketogenic diet, also and following the same steps you can fast for 18 and 20 hours, everything will always depend on your purpose, your preparation, and your body mainly.

Fasting as already mentioned, must be applied with absolute knowledge of what we want to achieve and the preconditions in which our body is to carry it out, in the case of weight loss, the main objective is to achieve ketosis and thus begin to lose that localized fat without having loss of muscle mass, we must also have knowledge of how to break the fast, and this step must be done gradually, that is to say, to break the fast they must consume slowly the foods, it is advisable to begin with a broth of bones for example, and is that with the practice of the fast also you can determine which are the possible foods that produce inflammation to you, since after having a period of time without consuming foods and to begin gradually to ingest them, you can determine if some of them produces discomfort to you, for example, or inflammation in your organism.

Whether for weight loss or any other purpose, it is necessary to remember that we must break the fast with a balanced diet and within the ketogenic diet because otherwise, everything achieved with fasting would be lost.

When we apply fasting in any of the cases explained above, one of the first things that occur is that the levels of sugar and insulin in the blood decrease, it is observed that it increases the body's response to insulin, which is the hormone that regulates blood sugar levels, therefore regulating these levels begins to burn that localized fat that we all want to eliminate from our body.

Fasting also increases the production of growth hormone, adrenaline, and glucagon, which are responsible for activating the mechanism of lipolysis, which is the combustion of fats, thus helping to eliminate body fat while preserving the muscles. It is a type of food in which there is no hunger, and excellent results are obtained.

After two to three weeks of limiting carbohydrate intake to less than 50 grams per day and applying fasting you start to observe how blood sugar levels fall, it is advisable to also consume salt in meals to prevent some of the side effects. When fasting is done there are periods of keto-adaptation that is generally achieved between two to four weeks, there are studies that classify the keto-adaptation in three phases, the short phase of adaptation that is achieved from 7 to 14 days, the medium phase that is achieved from 14 to 35 days of fasting, and the long phase of adaptation that is achieved from 2 to 12 months. In the process of keto-adaptation, what can be observed is a considerable decrease in symptoms caused by carbohydrate restrictions, when a keto-adaptation process is being carried out, the body feels more energetic, the body is already detoxified, and the changes and benefits in our body are beginning to be noticed.

Fasting has the particularity that can be chosen in an open way, that is, yourselves can choose what type of fast to choose, what type of food you should consume and when you should consume, this makes it a method to lose weight quite flexible, and in fact, by being able to be applied in this way and not be a strict diet has been achieved that more and more people are applying it successfully.

It is a good method to achieve slimming and increase fat burning and is that when the body reaches ketosis, the body is responsible for taking the fat accumulated from our body and thus burns the fat we have accumulated. In the case of training done on a fast, there are opinions that suggest that it is good to exercise on a fast because on a fast the body has fewer amounts of glucose and in this way it uses fat to acquire the energy demanded by exercise, in fact, there are studies that have shown that exercising on a fast burns more fat than doing it after eating. Although exercising on fasting is good, it is also recommended not to do high-intensity exercises. Again it is recommended that these practices are performed in a controlled manner by trained people. Not everyone can apply fasting, not everyone can exercise fasting, it is necessary to carefully evaluate the individual capacities of each person to implement these protocols, what is certain is that great benefits have been observed when applying them and that in the case of weight loss the results have been quite encouraging, moreover, all these methods to lose weight depend mainly on perseverance and planning to perform them, it is necessary and advisable to consume supplements, vitamins, minerals, electrolytes, in conjunction with the implementation of fasting and ketogenic diets.

CHAPTER 9: FOOD INCLUDED ON INTERMITTENT FASTING

In order to know what types or which foods are included or allowed when fasting, we must know what kind of fasting we will perform. However, the foods do not change a lot according to the fasting of our preference. So, we will give you an example of the food included in the 16/8 fasting

What is Intermittent Fasting 16/8 Based on?

This type of intermittent fasting is very simple and only consists of dividing our day "meal plan" in two, of which 8 hours will be in those we are allowed to eat, and 16 hours will be the hours in which our body will be fasting.

Usually, these 16 hours of fasting include the hours of sleep, so it is easier to do this without being fully aware of the time we spend fasting.

We can present a very simple case describing the lifestyle of a person who carries out this diet, this person in his intermittent diet 16/8 gets up at 8:00 AM to do their physical activity such as cardio for 45 minutes, then makes his first meal at 12:00 pm (from here starts the 8 hours) until 8 pm, when eats his dinner and after two hours goes to sleep. If we count his night hours, we can see that this person is able to take a light fast which is not reflected in such a heavy way.

One of the great advantages of this diet is the ease of adapting it to our lifestyle, so we do not become so complicated a task to be able to maintain a proper diet.

How Can I Organize My Intermittent Fasting Schedules?

How we will make our approach to the 16/8 method of the intermittent diet, we will propose a series of schedules with which we can govern ourselves initially, but these will always depend on our agenda and ability to fulfill them.

We will have as a first option the most used: This 8-hour diet starts from 10:00 in the morning and ends at 6:00 pm, entering a period of fasting from 6:00pm to 10: 00 am, thus having our 16 hours of fasting.

As a second option, we will have the previously explained where the first meal begins at 12:00 pm, having as last meal dinner at 8:00 pm.

As a third option, we have the case in which the first meal is at 1:00 pm, being the last meal at 9:00 pm.

Can Fasting Cause Hunger Attacks?

Many times the fear factor of people when fasting is the fear of "suffering from hunger," which generates anxiety so strong that they could end up eating even worse than they should.

Well, this is a myth, because at the moment each meal arrives we learn to enjoy more and we can even feel satisfied with each bite without having to exceed ourselves.

However, to avoid having such cravings during fasting hours, it is essential that each meal contains nutritious foods so that we can get that feeling of being satisfied. In case we come to present an episode of anxiety or craving the most advisable is to drink a glass of water or alternatively a vegetable broth to soothe a little, there will come the point at which we get used and can even favor us in complementing our food dishes.

Does Coffee Break the State of Fasting?

Up to now, no data has been found to confirm that drinking coffee can take us out of the fasting state. Even many experts include coffee in the diet or fasting regime (as long as this is coffee alone, without any "topping" or sugar)

However, there are cases of people who prefer to avoid coffee and resort to options such as homemade broths of vegetables, water and salt, sugarless gum, and even drink a lot of water. All this is acceptable as long as we avoid soft drinks (with or without sugar) and packaged juices.

Can I Eat Anything Once my Fasting Hours Are Over?

Once our fasting hours are over, the ideal is to eat (and drink) as healthily as possible, as it is useless to fast if we do not eat properly.

In the case of fasting, it is recommended to follow the Harvard dish model. What is this?

This is just one way to serve our food. It will be as follows: The main part of our plate (which will contain half of it) will be vegetables; a quarter will be carbohydrates, the other quarter will be meats (red or white such as fish, chicken) or legumes.

With this, we seek that the heaviest of our foods are vegetables and carbohydrates, and proteins are the companions of our meals.

Additionally, if we want a dessert, we recommend fruit, fruit salad, or yogurt, always avoiding those quick snacks that are not of natural origin.

What Foods Are Recommended for the Permitted Feeding Hours?

Really there is no diet by which we must regulate ourselves in a mandatory way since it is considered that with fasting, we are burning the necessary calories. However, it is always good to maintain a properly balanced diet so that these lost calories can be noticeable in the long term in our body.

Mostly it is recommended the consumption of fresh foods such as vegetables and fruits. This way, we are starting with a better lifestyle through food. The amounts of protein and even the same fresh food should be provided by a nutritionist as it will help us improve certain aspects based on what our body needs.

How Many Meals Per Day?

Usually, when making this type of diet, you have 2 or 3 main meals, and even in some cases, there are people who make a small snack (as long as it is within the hours in which the intake of food is allowed).

- If a person usually wakes up late, they can start the day with lunch, have a mid-afternoon mini snack and finally close with dinner.

There are other cases of morning people starting their day with a full breakfast, lunch, and dinner/snack.

Next, we are going to see an example of a menu that could serve us as a base to adapt our menu, according to our needs:

Intermediate Fasting 16/8: Morning Option

If you are one of those persons who start their day very early, you will need enough energy to perform in your daily tasks, so this is the option that can best suit you.

In this option, you will be able to eat food only from 10:00 am to 6:pm (18:00h), the rest of the time our body will be in a state of fasting:

- 7:00 am Start the day with tea, coffee, infusion, or water.
- 10:00 am First meal, full breakfast.
- 2:00 pm (14:00 hrs): Lunch
- 6:00pm (18:00 hrs): Snack or dinner
- 8:00 pm (20:00 hrs): In case of anxiety, hunger, or cravings, you can prepare a vegetable broth or some tea.

If you are one of those persons who love to sleep and start their day a little later than usual, you should be very attentive to what are your mealtimes and to be able to meet everything at the time, so this is the option that can best suit you.

In this option you will be able to eat only from 12:00 am to 8:pm (20:00h), the rest of the time our body will be in a state of fasting:

- 9:00 am Start the day with tea, coffee, infusion, or water.
- 12:00 am First meal; this must be a complete lunch to be able to contribute all the necessary energies.
- 3:00 pm (14:00 hrs): snack
- 6:00pm (18:00 hrs): dinner
- 8:00 pm (20:00 hrs): In case of anxiety, hunger, or cravings, you can prepare a vegetable broth or some tea.

HOW LONG IS IT RECOMMENDED TO CONTINUE WITH THE INTERMITTENT FASTING ROUTINE?

The most recommendable thing is to follow this regime until we obtain the changes that we look for to obtain in our organism and body. Nevertheless, we must not forget that also to obtain these results we have to exercise constantly.

Similarly, it is not totally forbidden that we can give ourselves a pleasure (dessert, pizza, hamburger, soda, etc.) from time to time.

We cannot forget an important complement. Do some physical activity:

In order to achieve the desired weight (and even physical endurance) is very important to exercise at least 3 times a week, so the effects of fasting will be more noticeable.

If we want to do physical activity during the 16 hours of fasting, we can only take the following:

- Water
- Tea
- Infusions
- Coffee (no sugar)
- Vegetable broth (preferably shredded)

If you are very anxious, you may be able to calm your anxiety with sugar-free gum.

These drinks are okay as long as they don't contain sugar, sweeteners, vegetables, milk, or anything else that may contain calories.

So, when fasting, there is no forbidden food or a list of food that is allowed, but the food you eat after fasting will mean a lot to get the results you are looking for. In order to get the best results, it is strongly recommended to eat using the keto diet after fasting. We will discuss how these two methods are related in the following chapter.

CHAPTER 10: INTERMITTENT FASTING AND KETO DIET

The ketogenic diet, as we appreciated in previous chapters, has a great number of benefits for the organism. It is a very popular feeding method nowadays and in which the fundamental purpose for which it is used is to lose weight.

As we already know with the low-carbohydrate diet, without consuming processed sugar and other conditions that carry the keto eating plan, different levels of ketosis can be reached, which finally, for people who do it in an adequate and disciplined way, is what they hope to reach.

Added to this, is intermittent fasting, which is a complement to the keto diet because it has been proven that people who apply it together reach ketosis faster.

Now, some people have managed to confuse this plan with the fact of going hungry, and in fact it is not recommended that this happens, to reach the levels of ketosis it is not necessary to go hungry or consume the already known "keto cravings", the fundamental thing is to avoid carbohydrate-rich foods such as cereals, sugars, legumes, rice, potatoes, sweets, of course, juices and most fruits.

The standard ketogenic diet is a diet plan that is characterized by being very low in carbohydrates, with a moderate intake of protein and high in fat. It normally contains 75% fat, 20% protein, and only 5% carbohydrates. As we already know if all these requirements are met blood sugar levels can be reduced and insulin levels too, and this way there will be a transition in the metabolism of the body in which carbohydrates are replaced as energy source for the body by fats and ketones, thus reaching the main objective which is "ketosis". When the insulin levels fall, ketones are manufactured, and this can be noticed in the second, third or fourth week. This period is known as Keto-adaptation (KA). The body becomes dependent on sugar as the main fuel ((glycogen) to depend mainly on fat and for this to be achieved, we must overcome the keto-adaptation phase.

When we finally change our main fuel we are going to have an unlimited fuel for fat to which people with other types of diet do not have access, and on the other hand, we are going to have glycogen as a secondary fuel, And that is how our body must actually work, because we are able to store 2000kcal of glycogen but more than 1,000,000 kcal of fat safely so we can store energy for ourselves.

For a person who must consume 2000 kcal daily it is achieved with the keto diet in the following way:

70-80%, which are equivalent to 1400-1600 kcal of fat, 15-25%, which corresponds to 300-500 kcal of protein, 5% of carbohydrates, which corresponds to approximately 100 kcal. More or less, we would be talking about 150-170 grams of fat per day, 75-125 grams of protein per day, and 25 grams of carbohydrates per day approximately.

But all these amounts are easy to get if we eat naturally, if we get our meals to be based mainly on meat, fish especially oily fish, egg, cheese, cream, all kinds of vegetables and this opens a large window of food, mushrooms, nuts, seeds, MCT oil, coconut oil, olive oil preferably extra virgin, butter or ghee, fruits such as avocado, coconut, berries, strawberries, blueberries, blackberries,. Basically, eat unprocessed food and processed organic from natural preference, but each of us will be able to structure our eating plan in the way we consider most appropriate.

Within ketosis, we have the term known as "nutritional ketosis", which is nothing more than consuming foods that do not depend on fat or protein, in order to reach the metabolic state called ketosis, we simply must completely and absolutely eliminate sugar, wheat and its derivatives and lower to its minimum expression the simple carbohydrates, and eliminate in its entirety the complex carbohydrates, which are commonly known as processed foods, bread, pasta, hamburger, etc..

In this way what is going to happen is that in your organism the glucose reserves are going to be depleted, and the ketogenic bodies will begin to feed, to look for energies of that accumulated fat in your body that we so much want to eliminate and it is there where you begin to feel the ketogenic state or ketosis. In fact, a high fat-burner in a natural way is the intermittent fasting practiced in a responsible and supervised way. If it is applied correctly, the consumption of artificial burners that we find in the different national and international markets is not necessary, so it is only a matter of organization and discipline, and you will begin to experience all the changes in your body and in your health. An exact way to determine if you are already in Ketosis is with a simple blood test, currently in the same way that there are devices on the market that have the ability to measure blood sugar levels, there are also several brands that can measure the levels of ketones in your body, so you can acquire any of them and thus keep track and know when you have reached the optimal level of ketosis.

However, when you stop consuming sugar and carbohydrates, you will mainly start a detoxification process, as the body begins to eliminate all that amount of anti-nutrients that for so long have been allowed into your body and has also damaged your cellular environment. When this detoxification process begins, you will suffer a series of unfriendly symptoms known as " abstinence syndrome," in this case, you will begin to experience the following symptoms:

- Sleeping difficulties.
- Apathy and listlessness.
- Symptoms of depression.
- Irritable attitude.
- Appetite disturbances.
- Lethargy.
- Anxiety.
- Thirst.

All these symptoms mentioned are due to your body starts to suffer the " abstinence syndrome " because you have restricted your body of carbohydrates and sugars, but before the appearance of these symptoms we have some recommendations that you can do when you feel that way:

- Drink plenty of water,
- It is recommended to drink apple vinegar, prepared as follows, dilute one tablespoon of vinegar in 4 ounces of water each morning on an empty stomach.
- And the most important recommendation is to eat well, it is not necessary as previously recommended to go hungry. Since once this stage is over, everything will be easier.

The important thing is to eat within the allowed requirements, but without going hungry, in fact you will notice that once your body has finally been detoxified and cleaned, your body begins to change and you begin to learn to listen to your body, and this means that when you eat a food that is harmful or alters your cellular environment, it will indicate with discomfort that you should not eat that food. In addition, you will have better absorption of nutrients because your digestive system improves, being one of the most important benefits of this diet since the intestine is currently considered as the second brain.

Now, as for fasting, we already know all the benefits involved in applying it, and the most important is that it is a potential fat burner for our body, helps reduce cellulite, among other great benefits that we already know. But fasting means not to eat and the intermittent fasting means not to eat for a period of time. It could be daily, weekly or monthly as you wish to apply it.

What will break your fast? Food. Fasting will promote the autophagy or recycling process of damaged cellular components, and large benefits of fasting are directly related to autophagy. But this process occurs gradually and will depend on our particular organism. It will depend on each tissue whether neurons, liver, muscle, immune system, intestines, and yes, the whole body in general.

There are studies that relate exercise, diet, and fasting with autophagy. All this process takes time; the changes are not going to happen overnight. First, the body must go through a process of adaptation.

In autophagy, the cell needs energy, and with the implementation of fasting and in the absence of exogenous food, the destruction of damaged internal contents begins, and autophagy begins. In this case, the cells will devour or consume parts of themselves to eliminate viruses, bacteria and all the damage caused by cellular aging and at the same time, obtain fuel to improve their processes.

This process is fundamental for the organism because if it is not carried out, it will lead to inflammatory processes, infectious diseases, Alzheimer's, Parkinson's and cancer. The autophagy achieved or stimulated through fasting is an intelligent way for the body to detoxify itself in a natural way since the cells themselves know what they need and what they don't need for their growth and evolution. Intermittent fasting eliminates toxins, stimulates the immune system, regulates inflammation and promotes longevity.

Generally, the intermittent fast that is performed is 16-8, this method 16/8 is known as "Leangains" method, with this modality you will consume food for 8 hours, and you will fast for 16 hours. If you wish, you can include within the 16 hours of fasting the period of sleep, so that it is easier and bearable this period of intermittent fasting. If you apply it in this way the most common is to lengthen breakfast at noon or what would be lunch, and finally your second meal of the day corresponds to the dinner, at night before 8 pm. This is an easy way to apply intermittent fasting daily accompanied by the keto diet, and if you can also if you can add exercise, you will love the final results.

And it is that the intermittent fast is more than a simple restriction of calories, it also produces alterations in the hormones of our body so that they can make better use of their fat reserves. By lowering insulin levels produces a better burning of fat. The secretion of growth hormone increases and, therefore, accelerates the synthesis of protein and using the fat that is available as a source of energy. So that is not only burning fat, but it is also building muscle mass more quickly as if you consume as athletes do. What a wonderful piece of news, isn't it? all that your body is capable of doing naturally if you just take the time to eat properly.

Now, how we should break with that fast?, or how we will have break-fast?, and is that one of the classic ways to break the fast is with the famous "bone broth", preferably homemade, but an hour before breaking the fast is recommended to drink a glass of soda water; it can be with cinnamon or apple vinegar, salt or lemon, this drink will help you prepare your stomach digestive enzymes that have been without food for 16 hours with only water and coffee, if you consume this drink it is likely that the food can be absorbed without stomach problems and absorbing all the nutrients to the maximum. After this, we can consume the bone broth, which is a liquid food will not force our stomach to work with heavy food, but rather easy digestion apart from the bone broth is rich in fat, protein, and vitamins. And an hour later you can eat a plate of solid food under the requirements of the keto diet, which you already know widely, this is a way to break the fast in a way suitable for your body, and to quickly reach ketosis and autophagy.

CHAPTER 11: SPECIFIC BENEFITS FOR YOUR HEALTH

When we observe the normal functioning of human beings, we can see that the body feeds on glucose, which is the molecule that is generated by the consumption of carbohydrates and sugars, but an excessive consumption of them, could cause damage to our health, such as becoming diabetics, which is a disease that occurs when glucose is produced in excess, and the body is not able to use it, having an excess of glucose in the blood, so to speak, causing problems in our organs, also, an excess consumption of carbohydrates can generate overweight, leading us, in the long run to very serious diseases, such as could be, the diabetes mentioned above.

Therefore, it could be said that this way of eating is not the best for our body, since the consumption of carbohydrates, either in a normal amount, the organs of our body do not always interact well with glucose, because having high levels of it in our body, insulin levels are also increased, and it has direct implications on the functioning of our body, so that it could even alter our metabolism.

Due to these reasons, we managed to achieve the state of ketosis, which is a state of our body, in which in a normal state, is a large consumption of fat, segregating a molecule called ketone, being this the main source of food for our body, or better said, is a source of energy extremely efficient and good for our body, which can produce side effects, not necessarily bad.

This function is essential for personal survival, since because of this, people can have an alternate source of energy, since at the time we run out of glucose, the body will proceed to consume their energy reserves produced by the ketone, of course, this energy reserve is not infinite, because the same may last a few days, therefore, this process is very important to continue with brain function in an effective way, because the process of storing glucose is very ineffective in our body, for that reason, we prefer to do the ketogenic feeding, because our body evolved to survive for several days, perhaps even weeks, being this an extremely extreme case, because the person is already trained to do this, not anyone is able to do such a task. Therefore, we could say that the process of ketosis is responsible for ensuring that the brain is feeding properly, in the event that you do not have enough glucose to feed it, and does so, as we explained previously, through the deposits of fat.

We can see that ketones interact in a better way with our organs, especially with our brain, since with this combination, the processes of the same can be carried out in a more optimal way. And as we should know, or at least intuit it, the brain is the organ that consumes more energy, therefore, to have a good ketone-brain relationship, we can say that our body is able to work better than with glucose, and is not that our brain works with fat, no, but with the molecules that segregate the liver, product of high fat consumption and low carbohydrate consumption, therefore, the brain proceeds to work with the ketones, thus achieving a more efficient consumption of energy, moreover, we assume that you have suffered episodes in your life in which you feel exhausted, without the need to have done many exercises or many activities, a possible reason for this condition, is that your body is poorly alimented, because your body is not generating much glucose or is not processing it well, by this we mean, to having a high level of glucose in the blood, insulin levels rise, and people feel a certain tiredness, a palpable example is that when you eat a large plate of pasta, immediately after you feel tired and sleepy, this is due to the fact that your insulin levels are high, producing a state of heaviness in your body, but in the case that you do or practice another type of diet, you will feel more energy, furthermore, there are people who, with only the ketogenic diet, have managed to fast for long periods of time, without feeling short of energy, thus having a better performance of our body, concluding that our brain, when it sees the opportunity to feed on ketones produced by the consumption of fat, feels more energy, indeed, there are people who certify that when they changed their habits, they started to feel more energetic, and if this was not enough, they also felt better mentally focused, so we cannot say that this diet is not only responsible for losing weight but physically benefit our body.

But, we are going to go step by step, therefore we will explain little by little the benefits of the consumption of a good ketogenic diet for our body, which can even improve the state of the heart of our body, due to this reason, we invite you to migrate from food diet, of course, if you wish, since you will be able to observe in a fast way the improvement in your health.

As we already know, the ketogenic diet has many benefits for people who consume it, they can go from improving the brain condition of patients, to improve respiratory problems of people, for that reason, they are not only needed to lose weight but also for some pathologies that you may have and want to solve.

The first benefit that it provides us, is as well it is known, the decrease of the weight, this result is obtained thanks to that the keto diet, is in charge of burning the fat and in this process of burning it is entered into ketosis, coming this way to lose a great number of kilograms, obtaining a better health in the people who suffer from obesity. When achieving the goal of coming out of the obesity state, the following benefits can be obtained:

- Reduces the possibility of death, as obesity is the leading cause of death in the United States.
- The possibility of suffering from diseases such as cancer, diabetes, heart attacks, gallstones.
- Many people who are overweight feel a lot of depression because of the shape of their body, and when they get out of it, these people improve their mental health, thus increasing their quality of life.
- There are many people who, because they are overweight, do not sleep very well for different reasons, but the main reason is sleep apnea, which is a cause closely related to overweight, which can cause high blood pressure or even heart attacks.

As we can already see, reducing our body weight can significantly improve our quality of life since overweight affects us in many areas of health, and not only the visual that is also important, but it can affect us so much that it can lead to death.

We can also find a direct relationship between the ketogenic diet and the health of the heart, because as we explained previously, this type of food, allows a rapid loss of body fat index, therefore, allow us to quickly lose weight, because it burns fat in an exaggerated form so to speak, thus achieving a more than considerable reduction in cardiovascular risks, because they have a close relationship with obesity, because if the person is obese, then it has more chances of having heart disease, coupled with this, being obese implies that you have a high blood pressure, which could cause a heart attack, which can be fulminant or not. On the other hand reduces the amount of cholesterol in our body, which indicates that we have a large amount of fat in our blood, and having such a condition can also cause some of our arteries to block, which can also lead to a heart attack. For these reasons, we recommend doing the low-carbohydrate diet, so as to achieve reduce these pathologies and clean our body of fats found in our blood, thus achieving a better protection of our blood system thereby preventing this type of disease, otherwise, also when practicing the ketogenic diet, we achieve a cell cleaning in our blood, throwing harmful toxins into our body, due to the process of increased autophagy, which, as we said previously cleanses our body, and there is nothing better than having the body clean, because having our body so, we can begin to see it work better or improve its functioning by cleaning ourselves internally, since our body will work as new, without any impediment. But said all this, and explained that this diet reduces cholesterol and all of the above, you may wonder: why make a high-fat diet low cholesterol if I was banned from fried chicken, and this is no more than fried protein? Well, it is not that all fats are good, on the contrary, there is nothing more harmful than some fried foods, for that reason it is not a very good practice to eat them, but what is true, is that you can consume many fats, as long as they are good fats from nature, such as avocado fat, or natural peanut butter.

As if that were not enough, the keto diet, not only helps the heart, but to an accumulation of other organs, another very important one, I would not know if I could tell you that the most important in the body, but if the one that consumes the most energy, such as the brain, the first thing we can say about the relationship of the ketogenic diet with the brain, is that in one of the first cases that the keto diet was implemented, it was in a patient suffering from epilepsy, which indicates that the patient suffered from constant convulsions, and by prescribing a diet low in carbohydrates, but higher in fat, a considerable improvement could be observed. Then, we can say that studies have been done on people who suffer from epilepsy, and the results conclude that this diet does help them, but it, is recommended more frequently to children, since it is easier to guide a child who is going to eat or not, and also the brain of the adult is already fully formed. The results are very positive, since at least half of the children to whom the test was applied, stopped suffering epileptic seizures, and another amount, even more than fifty percent, since here we also count those who did not suffer their epileptic seizures anymore, but those who had their frequency of epileptic seizures considerably reduced, therefore, we cannot be one hundred percent conclusive, saying that it ends with epilepsy or something like that, but there is something that we can say, and it is that the results are hopeful for a bright future, in the field of epilepsy. Also, the same diet can be used for those who suffer from Alzheimer's, since it is a degenerative disease, which causes people to gradually lose their memory, until the time comes when they can remember almost nothing, becoming so complicated the situation that can lead to the death of patients with the disease. We can say that the results are positive, it is because first, the experiments carried out on animals, were positive, since the mice which had certain brain degeneration, were given ketogenic food, and it was possible to obtain, first, that they managed to regenerate parts of their brains, and second, because it has also been achieved that the ketogenic food manages to improve the connections between the axons and dendrite, thus obtaining better communication between neurons, obtaining a brain more capable of performing any kind of tasks.

So, what we can say with this, is that we recommend you feed yourself with ketogenic food, because as you could have seen, not only helps us to reduce our weight, but we can improve a large accumulation of health conditions, improving the lives of our heart, improving our respiratory system or even reactivating some brain connections.

It is important to highlight the fact that the food used in the keto diet, such as fish and other seafood, has a lot of omega 3 and other components that are scientifically proven to have positive effects on brain functioning, performance, and memory.

CHAPTER 12: SLEEP, STRESS, AND MINDSET

Have you ever felt so stressed that you couldn't sleep? Many times those sleeping difficulties or insomnia are caused naturally in response to the levels of stress we may be under; in fact, sometimes, when we have trouble falling asleep, they can cause stress.

It is known that our mind has immense power when it is not calm, it directly affects the body, and it may be difficult for us to calm both in this type of situation.

Since we are young, we have used the word to say that we are stressed, but what is stress really?

We can define stress as the set of physiological reactions that are presented to us when we are suffering a state of nervous tension caused by various situations, whether anxiety, overwork, traumatic situations to which we have been exposed.

In this way, stress is directly associated with emotional distress and body tension. These when they increase their levels of excitement, which alert the body to prepare to face the possible danger to which we submit.

DIFFERENT TYPES OF STRESS

- Common Stress: They are the natural reactions that occur in our organism to certain situations, which we can define as stressful. Many times these types of stress are anxieties about something we are going to be under, and this natural reaction can help us overcome such situations.
- Workplace stress: This happens when the demands on our work environment are so huge that they cause us to collapse into harmful emotional and physical reactions to which our ability to solve a problem is not possible to solve.
- Pathological stress: This occurs when the stress we have is presented in an intense way for a prolonged period, which could cause us psychological and physical problems, causing anxiety crisis, crying crisis, depression, and many other physical alterations that turn this into chronic and constant stress.
- Post-traumatic stress: This is the stress that occurs after a person has lived through an event that significantly affected them, whether it was a traffic accident or a natural disaster. As a consequence of this trauma, the person often has thoughts that cause

terror. This type of stress occurs at any age but is mostly the result of childhood experiences.

Many times, the way in which we see ourselves in the world can influence these reactions of the body (just as the mind can betray us and make the situation look much worse, generating more anxiety).

This is why if we feel stressed or not, has a direct relationship with how we perceive things, for example, imagine that we have a very common case of everyday life which could be leading us to very high levels of stress:

In this case, we have to pay a household utility bill for $100, and we have two cases:

1. A person who has $1,000 in his account and pays that bill does not affect his budget.
2. A person who has $60 in his account and pays that bill would cost him a little bit because he would have to collect a little more and put aside any extra problems that affect his budget.

In these cases, we could observe how one person would find this situation totally normal, while another person could generate very great anguish and perceives more significantly the problem that is presented because his ability to evaluate the resources and face the problem could have a great impact on their mood.

If we look at stress as a way of trying to balance the demands of life and the resources we have to deal with it, we have two options:

1. Reduce the demands we perceive
2. Seek ways to increase our available resources.

It is important to emphasize that not always resources are limited to a monetary value, our resources could also make references to cognitive things such as improving our behavior, lifestyle, a way of thinking, skills to control our emotions, take control of some situation, have faith and even physical aspects such as improving our endurance and energy.

If we feel that we are facing a stress episode, we must ask ourselves the following questions in order to find a possible immediate solution; what is the factor that generates stress? What are the resources I have to solve this problem? How can I apply these resources to the solution of my problem?

Many times we focus more on the problem without taking into account that we have the solution in our hands. That is why before altering ourselves, we must think coldly about why the situation is happening, and in this way, we will be avoiding a worse result.

STRESS IN OUR BODY

Our body reacts to stress when the hormones that cause it are released; these cause our body to be attentive to any problem that might occur, this causes our body muscles to tension and thus progressively increase our heart rate.

This type of reaction could be interpreted as the way in which our body protects itself from any approaching danger and can even help us make quick decisions in any situation. The problem occurs when chronic stress occurs because our body will remain alert to any event even if we are not close to danger, and in the long term, could significantly affect our health.Chronic stress may cause us:

- Acne
- Menstrual problems
- High Blood Pressure
- Cardiac insufficiency
- Depression or anxiety
- Obesity

In addition to directly affecting health, it can influence our daily activities, or physical problems that we don't realize are caused by stress. These can be:

- Headaches.
- Lack of energy or concentration.
- Diarrhea.
- Constipation.
- Poor memory.
- Trouble sleeping.
- Sexual problems.
- Discomfort in the stomach.
- Need to use alcohol to feel temporarily distracted.
- Weight loss or gain

Sleeping is one of the resources which help to decrease stress in a considerable way, it helps us to cognitive processes such as good memory, concentration, and attention, it helps to the good psychological and emotional functioning since many times when a person does not rest enough he is in a bad mood and in this way he expresses his bad attitude towards the world.

Sleeping properly helps us recharge physical energy, improve injuries, and even growth.

Sleep is influenced by the body clock system and the dream controller. These are responsible for determining when to rest and for how long we should do it or for how long our body needs it.

If we have the correct functioning of our system, the one in charge of promoting the state of sleep will have power over our alert system every night. Unlike if we get to have a very high level of stress when resting, our system that is responsible for promoting the alerts of our body will have greater power over the system that promotes sleep, causing insomnia or difficulties to fall asleep.

Ideal advice to reduce the levels of stress that we may present when we go to bed to sleep:

If you feel too anxious to be able to promote sleep, you can get out of bed, drink a glass of water and try to relax your mind.

Plan a relaxing hour before going to bed: It is important that before going to bed, we have an hour to devote ourselves to bathing, relaxation stretching, and even reading. These simple exercises can relax our body from any problem that we have presented in the day.

The bed is a place to rest: It is important to avoid any type of activity that generates stress (tasks, work, fighting).

ADVICE TO BE ABLE TO LOOK FOR EASY SOLUTIONS TO OUR WORRIES

- Develop routines and habits: Performing physical activities and even eating a healthy diet can help our mind to clear and even improve our body clock.
- Self-care: It is important to spend time doing any type of activity that helps us mentally and makes us feel good. Many times we try to solve a problem without feeling good, and this is very important because it affects us emotionally and we will not have the energy to deal with another problem.
- Knowing our personal strengths: It is important to know the way we see ourselves. In this way, our problem-solving abilities could increase significantly when we know what we are capable of facing.
- Relaxation: It is important from time to time to take relaxation breaths to purify our body and connect it with the mind. A clean mind can think more clearly to an overwhelmed mind.

- Connect with others: It is important to receive support, and we achieve this by surrounding ourselves with our loved ones, so we know that we are not alone against the world. Many studies indicate that surrounding ourselves with loved ones can have a great influence on our physical and psychological health.

TIPS TO LESSEN OUR WORRIES:

Organization: It is important to dedicate at least one hour a day to be able to take care of everything that could worry us or could become a worry in the future. In this way, we will be able to obtain a better level of relaxation at night. It is advisable to write down everything. In this way, we do not overlook anything, and so we slowly go thinking about how to solve them (either present problem, something that has not happened or that we imagine a possible scenario which will not exist).

Thought: Our mind is a powerful weapon and from it can depend on our state of mind and even what we are capable of doing, to be able to do this we just have to put aside the negative thoughts and concentrate on the positive ones.

Many times we get involved in a negative scenario believing that we will never get out of that gap, but the reality is that you can, and everything depends on us, let's put the concerns aside and deal with it without fear of failing or at least trying.

Organizing our time: This is a very effective way to prevent future stress. Organizing our priorities is the most important thing because we avoid overlooking something and being always in order we can perform our daily tasks much faster.

Communication: Communicating our concerns or asking for some help is never too much. We do not know if we have a problem, and another subject has the solution (as the very known phrase states: Two heads think better than one). When we reduce the number of demands we have, our stress levels decrease dramatically.

Identify and communicate how we feel: Another effective way to prevent future stress may be to identify how we are feeling at that moment, whether we are going through a difficult time, or have had a discussion that may upset us. In these cases, it is advisable to go to a specialist, a friend or write our feelings on a piece of paper.

At This Point, We Must be Asking Ourselves: How Does This and the Keto Diet Relates? As we have seen before, it is well known that in order to follow a diet, we must adapt ourselves and our body to certain habits to which we may not have been used to. This will always be the key when it comes to any kind of diet because if we do not have the right mentality, we will not succeed in trying to adapt our body to it.

As human beings, we will always follow a pattern that has never failed since we were very small. Whenever we discover something new (in this case the keto diet), we get excited and set out to meet every goal needed to achieve the goal we have set for ourselves; over time we will notice the changes we have obtained as a result of the effort to accomplish certain rules. The problem comes when we have reached this objective, and we stop obeying strictly the rules (which led us to this objective).

In the case of the keto diet, we will need to strictly comply with all the steps, since in this way our body will begin to make certain changes and will need a period of adaptation to be able to receive these changes in a good way.

Many times, people who try to do this diet fail to see the promising results that everyone talks about doing the keto diet and enter a state of despair and stress. Why does this happen, this is for the simple reason that these people do not start with the right mentality, this could apply to any type of diet or feeding regime.

Through the following steps, we will achieve a good motivation and guidance to maintain the right mentality at the time of making this diet (or any other):

STEP 1: START WITH WHAT YOU HAVE

Many times when you start a diet, you feel motivated and start buying food based on a dietary plan that your body has not adapted to.

In most cases, when a person starts a diet or a strict diet is in order to lose weight, which is why it is considered very important to take it easy as you can not change habits drastically without consequences.

The process of our body to adapt to new habits should be gradual, if we start with what we have, we will gradually decrease the foods that do not suit us (as indicated by our specialist in nutrition), and thus our body will be able to assimilate these changes and release the old habits.

If we allow our body to assimilate these changes, we can see how the results are taking place by themselves, such as weight loss and improvement of some aspects of our health and even physical aspects. Unlike if we force our body to a drastic change, which can bring negative consequences such as weight gain or hormonal imbalance.

It is important to remember that the limits can only be set by ourselves, and it depends on how things work. Changes are always good as long as we accept them in a healthy way to ensure the basis for the success of our diet.

So if I do this correctly and start with what I have at home to change my diet, am I going to be successful with this diet?

As we mentioned earlier, before starting a diet, you must go to a nutritionist, and from here, we are going to enter into a kind of experiment in which we can evaluate whether this new style of feeding suits us or not.

Why an experiment? We can say that we submit ourselves to an experiment because we will not know if it will be successful and the diet will adapt to us effectively or cause negative effects, this is a risk to which we must be prepared, and we will begin with what we have to gain confidence as we get to know ourselves better.

It won't matter what level of physical condition we have or our daily routine of eating habits, as long as we feel willing to do something, it will come naturally; don't try hard to buy foods that may not be to your liking. Know yourself, and in this way, the other steps will be easy.

STEP 2: ENJOY YOUR FOOD

This step is directly related to step 1 because when we start with what we have in our kitchen, in a certain way are the foods we like and enjoy, if we eat healthily and at the same time feel comfortable with it. A diet will stop calling diet to become a habit.

Many times we fail because we have the mental chip that a diet is based on foods that we will not enjoy and will let us starve, this is false, we can not force ourselves to eat food that we do not tolerate, although it is clear that not everything will always be to our liking, we must take a good balance and not lean to just the extremes.

We should not be alarmed by this of new foods because it may be that as our system adapts to our new habit, our tastes will also change. At first, it may be very frustrating to put aside many of the foods to which we were used to, but instead of tying ourselves to a non-existent torment, we can go balancing the foods we like and those we don't to make our palate get used to.

It is important that we do not see the change of food as a punishment since, in this way, it can be much more complicated to adapt to a new diet. A change must be something exciting, something that intrigues us; we should not be predisposed to the unknown since the keto diet has many food alternatives that may be in accordance with us.

How can I make the process of adapting to new healthy foods easier if I like to eat unbalanced?

First, we must choose which style of keto diet we are going to follow according to our habits and willingness to respect them, followed by this we adapt the foods according to our tastes.

WHAT HAPPENS IF I DO NOT LIKE ANY FOOD INCLUDED IN THE DIET AND I CANNOT EAT IT?

Nothing at all will happen. We can easily look for an alternative food to replace the one we do not like. With this, we are not looking to change our taste buds, but we are looking for a healthier lifestyle. We must allow ourselves to enjoy the process and the changes, so we can embrace the results (weight loss, hormone regulation, etc.) in a more positive way.

I really like sweets and junk food, can it be the right diet for me?

Here arises the big problem that can suffer 50% of people who want to start the keto diet and do not dare, we know that we will accept a new challenge to which we must make certain sacrifices, among them is that, put aside the sweets and reduce them. This could be considered the only major sacrifice we can make when we start in keto.

It may cost us a little more to adapt to these kinds of changes, as it is not something that is achieved overnight. But we can make sure that by changing our mentality, we can succeed in everything we set out to do (even in the keto diet).

STEP 3: WE CAN DO IT

As mentioned above, it is very normal for us to be motivated when discovering or starting a new diet, and we want to get to the results that other people have gotten through this routine.

Many times these testimonials come with a marketing image to attract more people or consumers, so we will see photos that we could think and say are "perfect" and that we want to get to that point, the goal is not to give up.

Many times people are discouraged and feel they are failing because they have idealized that they will get the same results as other people who have told their experience with the diet, not all bodies react in the same way, there are people who may take a little longer and there are people to whom the results will be noticed instantly, but the key is persistence.

Once we have focused on how the diet should work our way, we can see another picture. Many times the road to the goal can be complicated, but the important thing is to keep insisting (in a healthy way), the best thing we could do is to tell our own version of how we take the diet to stay with the doubt of. How would the keto diet have worked for me?

This step is directly related to trust since we must be able to understand that we are capable of accomplishing anything as long as we are insistent and follow the rules properly. If we start a new project with the mentality that we may not be able to achieve it, we are complicating the road to success.

This is why we must mentally prepare ourselves to achieve success with keto, it may sound like an easy task, but in many cases, it can be complicated because, as we mentioned before, we are looking for "quick results" only for it, there is a long way to achieve it.

Once we have gone through those three steps, we should be or getting used to the keto diet. As we mentioned a lot of times in the previous chapter, this diet has a lot of benefits regarding the brain, health, and organs of the body. This new habit will help us to feel a bit less stressed because our body will perform better. We will have more confidence in ourselves. Hence we will be able to face the troubles easily. As the stress is reduced, and our body is on a perfect balance, sleeping will also improve, since no illness or pain or weakness will interrupt our sleep.

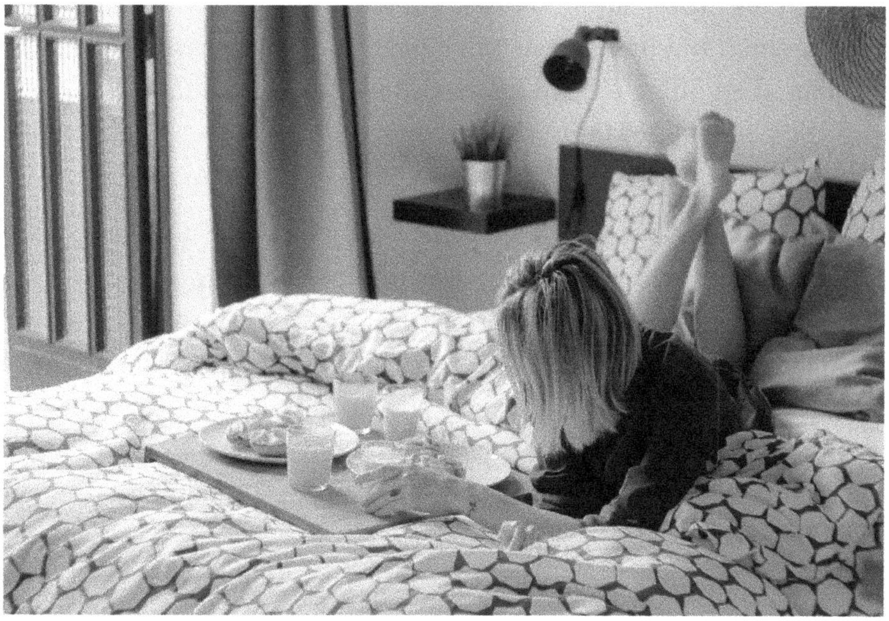

CHAPTER 13: LIFESTYLE AND DAILY ROUTINE

When we talk about the ketogenic diet, we want more than a diet to be implemented as a discipline and as a lifestyle, since in the case of the ketogenic diet, the long-term changes are those that have an important impact on our health.

When we apply this feeding method to our lifestyle while we start with the metabolic transition and the detoxification process where the body will seek to eliminate all the anti-nutrients we have ingested, we must constantly maintain this discipline so that we can finally clean our cellular environment and when this cellular environment is cleaned and healed it is very important to maintain this eating plan because the moment we return to consume anti-nutrients we return to damage our digestive system and therefore our cellular environment.

That is why it is advisable not to see it in a circumstantial way but rather as a lifestyle where we are learning little by little how to feed ourselves. We will get to know our body, and we will realize that our own body will indicate to us which foods do us harm or which ones we tolerate more and which ones we do not.

If we plan this lifestyle with a routine that we apply daily, it can be made easier to apply, we can plan our menus, and once we acquire experience it is easier for us to program the daily food plan, depending on the disposition of time you have, how you want to make the ketogenic diet if you want to take along with intermittent fasting and exercise, as in fact is commonly recommended to reach faster levels of ketosis and maintain these high levels of energy in our body.

Although many people now think that fat is harmful to health, it happens that with this lifestyle and fat intake we can turn off the fat-storage hormone and thus reprogram our genes to lose weight and burn fat, you are going to notice how the cravings and the desire to eat are reduced because you feel constantly satiated, so not only are you going to lose the kilograms you want, but also, as we have mentioned several times, to improve your health and it is that this should be your main objective and the one that pushes you to take this keto diet as a lifestyle.

The most important ingredient in any meal plan, as the word says is planning, because if we plan, we are not going to be tempted to make bad decisions that may be unhealthy in the end. This is why one of the recommendations we want to make is that at weekends you should take some time to do your weekly planning, your weekly menu, which you can probably alter during the week but to have a more orderly plan you can evaluate what you are going to consume based on the goal you want to achieve.

Start by organizing the dinners, which always turns out to be the most difficult thing to plan, manage, for example, two or three types of vegetables, with a source of proteins complemented of healthy fats always. If you can, add a rich and nutritious salad of vegetables, that way you are arming options of the menu for your week, in the case that your daily life allows it.

The same thing happens with breakfast, you can organize it in a planned way, you can even repeat them without any problem in several opportunities or add other contours to them, assuming that breakfasts are made, because in most cases the ketogenic diet is combined with the known intermittent fast and if it is there, breakfast is suppressed in most cases.

As you can notice everything is a matter of order and planning to make this meal plan a lifestyle, because only then you can get results for longer, and you will notice that as the days go by when you feel energetic, encouraged and in very good health you will not want to leave this lifestyle and your body will thank you.

CHAPTER 14:
KETO RECIPES FOR A GOOD FASTING

We already know the benefits that intermittent fasting brings to our health. We know that it helps to deal with stress and fatigue, delays the signs of aging, helps in the process of hormonal regulation, prevents diseases, improves fat metabolism, controls appetite, and achieves a longer time of autophagy or what is also known as cellular self-regulation.

Fasting helps to control appetite, so when we apply intermittent fasting, it is very easy to carry out a ketogenic diet.

The most important thing about intermittent fasting is that we must eat to break it and the first thing is to consider that as we have so many hours without eating food is not recommended that our first meal is very heavy, but rather it is recommended to break the fast with a liquid diet, and nothing is better than doing it with a broth of bones.

BONE BROTH

Ingredients:

- 1 kg of red beef bones fed on grass.
- Coriander, onion.
- 6 cloves of garlic.
- Salt to taste (preferably Himalayan salt.)
- Apple vinegar.
- Water

Steps to follow:

1. In a large pot place the bones and enough water leaving about 4 to 5 centimeters to the top of the pot and add the coriander to taste and half chopped onion, only to taste the boiling. Also, add 2 tablespoons of vinegar.
2. Let it rest without lighting the fire for about 20 to 30 minutes as the acid in the vinegar helps the nutrients in the bones become more available.
3. Add enough salt to taste and let cook for about two hours covered, over low heat, and we are alert not to dry our broth
4. It is important to check the broth and remove the foam that is formed above.
5. In the remaining 30 minutes, add more coriander and stir.

MEDALLIONS OF BEEF TENDERLOIN WITH COCONUT

The fusion of the coconut with the meat is an excellent mixture. This is a highly recommended recipe. Coconut, in turn, is an important ally in the ketogenic diet and in intermittent fasting.

Ingredients:

- 1 kg of beef tenderloin, preferably from grass-fed animals.
- 3 spoonfuls of coconut oil.
- 2 cloves of garlic.
- 1 sweet pepper
- 1 large onion.
- 500 ml coconut milk.
- 2 spoonfuls of ground thyme.
- Chicken consommé.
- Pepper to taste.
- Sea salt.

Steps to follow:

1. Let's start seasoning the beef tenderloin with the consommé, a little salt, and pepper, add to taste, and then let it rest for a period of two hours in the refrigerator.
2. Then in a large pot over medium heat, add the coconut oil, and the whole garlic is fried, and when the garlic is browned, we take them out, so we season the oil.
3. Now add the beef tenderloin and seal on both sides. This process can take about 5 minutes.
4. Then we will finely chop the onion along with the paprika and add the thyme and stir several times for flavors to stick.
5. Add the coconut milk, salt, and cover. Let it boil for 30 to 40 minutes or until the loin feels cooked and soft.
6. The sauce will thicken and take a golden tone; this dish should be served hot.

This dish can be served with cauliflower rice or with salads.

CAULIFLOWER CAKE

Ingredients:

- 2 cups cauliflower

- 400 grams of ground beef.
- 4-5 slices of Mozzarella cheese.
- ½ onion
- Sea salt to taste.
- ½ cup whipping cream.

Steps to follow:

1. First, we wash the cauliflower very well. We will add in a pot enough water to boil add the cauliflower for a few minutes until it cooks, it is not recommended to cook for long vegetables, the idea is to cook it al dente. After it is ready, we submerge it in ice water for a few minutes to cut the cooking. Then we strained and reserved.
2. In a frying pan, we are going to fry the onion and the ground meat; we add salt to the taste, pepper if we like.
3. In the blender, pour the whipping cream, salt and add the cauliflower little by little.
4. This way, you will get a kind of mashed potatoes when you finish blending all the cauliflower.
5. In a lasagne mold, we are going to distribute the ground meat that we prepared previously. We are going to spread it uniformly by all the tray.
6. On top of this layer, we are going to add the cream that we made with the cauliflower and, finally, a layer with the slices of Mozzarella cheese. We are going to place everything in a uniform way.
7. Finally, we take it to the oven for 15 minutes until the cheese melts.

When we practice intermittent fasting, one of the advantages we acquire with time and discipline is that we have no appetite because our body acquires a lot of energy. And we are going to feel that. That's why the food that complements fasting is simple but enough for you to feel satisfied. The advisable thing is always to choose natural products, and of good quality, in addition to evaluating the nutritional contributions, the vegetable has that you are going to consume for example. At first, it is probably a bit tedious, but as you acquire experience and knowledge, it becomes easier to organize food plans because one of the objectives we want to achieve is to improve the health of our body.

CHAPTER 15: RECIPES FOR BREAKFAST AND SNACKS

In a world as dynamic, and as fast as the actual, we can not go around without breakfast, or being hungry over there, unless we are doing some fasting or something like that, as being in a diet already prepared, but in the event that you are not fasting, you cannot walk on your day without breakfast, much less with hunger, for that reason, we recommend, as long as you can, to have breakfast, since this is one of the most important meals of the day, and why not? Sometimes eat a snack at mid-morning or in the afternoon.

BREAKFAST

In this book, we will share two recipes to have a good breakfast, which can feed you adequately, the other breakfasts that you want to eat, you are going to create them, since one of the benefits of the ketogenic diet, is that the recipes are extremely simple.

KETO OMELET

This is a recipe extremely simple and quick to make, many of the people who have prepared such a recipe, say it is better than the classic omelet served in restaurants, because it is spongy and very rich, it allows us to have a variety of ingredients in our omelet, without the need to spend so much money, because we can add cheese, ham, paprika, and onion to our omelet, and it is perfect for people who have a very rushed life, as it not only gives us a good amount of energy to do all our activities but also allows us not to waste much time in the kitchen.

Now, the ingredients of the omelet that we are going to recommend are the following:

- Six eggs.
- Two tablespoons of sour cream, or can also be whipped cream, to taste of the consumer.
- Salt to taste.
- Pepper to taste.
- Three ounces of grated cheese, no matter the type of cheese, can be smoked, gouda, the important thing is that it contains fat.
- Two ounces of butter.

- Five ounces of smoked ham cut into squares.
- Half medium onion, chopped into very small squares.
- Half green bell pepper, which has to be chopped into very thin strips.

It should be noted that you can add the ingredient you want, in addition to the proportions that were supplied here, are an estimate, you can add more or less to it.

After having the ingredients ready, we can proceed to the preparation of our recipe, in the following steps:

- Pour the six eggs and the cream over a bowl, then mix until you have a homogeneous and creamy mixture.
- Add salt and pepper.
- Add half of the grated cheese, after this, proceed to beat the mixture well again.
- Then, in a frying pan, melt the butter over medium heat, it is important that it is at this heat so that the butter does not burn.
- Pour the ham over the pan when the butter is melted, and proceed to fry the ham, paprika, and onions for a while, or until the onions are golden brown.
- Pour the eggs and cream mixture into the frying pan where the ham and onion were, then fry until the omelet is cooked.
- Reduce the heat for a while, and pour the rest of the grated cheese over the omelet, waiting for it to melt.
- Fold it.
- Take it out of the frying pan and cut it in half.

As you can see, the recipe is extremely simple. The same does not consume much time, less than ten minutes for sure, therefore, this recipe is very productive for people who have a very fast life, thus achieving a healthy and complete breakfast in less than ten minutes.

SCRAMBLED EGGS WITH FETA CHEESE

This is an extremely simple recipe, which allows people who do not have much experience cooking, to eat very healthy, very nutritious, and very rich in a short time, since the time it should take you to make this recipe is about ten or fifteen minutes. In addition to this, scrambled eggs can be added to any type of ingredients you want, such as bacon, ham, or even spinach. The ingredients for our recipe are as follows:

- Four eggs.
- Two good tablespoons of whipped cream, thick.

- Two tablespoons of butter.
- Four ounces of spinach.
- A finely chopped garlic clove.
- A quarter of shredded feta cheese.
- Salt to taste.
- Pepper to taste.
- Four ounces of bacon.

After we have all the ingredients ready, we can proceed to start with the preparation.

1. In a bowl, beat the eggs and cream until they are homogeneous and well creamy.
2. Cook the bacon until well cooked.
3. In a frying pan, melt the butter over medium heat.
4. After the butter is melted, proceed to add the other ingredients, such as spinach and garlic, wait until the spinach is cooked, you will notice if the spinach is withered.
5. Add the bacon to the pan, and add salt and pepper to taste.
6. Pour over the frying pan, the mixture that contains the eggs, then wait until the edges of the frying pan begin to bubble, at this time, with the help of a spoon, stir from outside to inside, repeating the process until they are cooked.
7. Remove the scrambled eggs from the pan, and add the feta cheese, in this part, you can also add a little more bacon if you choose.

As you can see, this recipe is extremely simple, so you can do it many times, you can change it and have different breakfasts for your whole week, just pretend you are the chef.

SNACKS

These foods are important when you've already eaten, but gives you a little hunger, for that reason, people turn to snacks, but in the case of those who do not have a ketogenic diet, they can go to some Cheetos or Doritos, but in our case, that we are with another type of food, we will have our nutritious snacks.

CHEESE CHIPS

This recipe is extremely simple, and you don't need many ingredients to make them since all you need is cheese and paprika.

The ingredients are exactly as follows:

- Eight ounces of cheese, whether yellow, gouda, cheddar, provolone.
- Half a spoonful of paprika.

As we can see, the ingredients are more than basic, to have our fantastic snack. The preparation is as follows.

1. Preheat oven to 400°F.
2. Grate the cheese of your preference, and place it in small piles on a tray to put it in the oven, it is important to say that the tray must be lined with parchment paper. It is important to leave enough space so that when they melt, the piles of cheese do not touch.
3. Sprinkle the paprika over the grated cheese.
4. Bake for about ten to eight minutes until you see that the cheese is ready, do not let the cheese burn.
5. Let them cool and serve.

As you can see, this snack is extremely simple, and you don't need many ingredients, and so are the great majority of the snacks in the ketogenic diet. Therefore, we don't tell you more and go to the kitchen to see how delicious this recipe is.

CHAPTER 16:
LUNCH AND DINNER RECIPES

These other foods continue to be vital to our organism, to the point that we consider them to have the same importance as breakfast.

LUNCHES

After breakfast, between the twelve noon (12:00 pm) and the one o'clock (1:00 pm), we proceed to eat this meal, so that it continues to give us energy for the rest of the day.

KETO TACOS

This recipe is very simple since we are supplanting the carbohydrates of the cookie of the tacos, with cheese, which is an amazing idea and simple to make.

The ingredients are as follows:

- Two cups of cheddar cheese, gouda, grated parmesan.
- A spoonful of extra virgin olive oil.
- An onion chopped in small squares.
- Three cloves of garlic finely chopped.
- A pound of ground beef.
- Half a spoonful of ground cumin.
- Half a spoonful of paprika.
- Salt to taste.
- Black pepper to taste.
- Sour cream.
- Avocados, chopped in small squares.
- Fresh cilantro.
- Freshly chopped tomatoes, in small squares.

The next steps are as follows:

1. Preheat the oven to 400°F, and line the baking tray with the parchment paper.
2. Serve the cheese on the tray as piles, and make sure they have some distance so that when melted, the piles of cheese do not stick.

3. Bake until the cheese bubbles and begins to brown.
4. Let cool for about six minutes.
5. Then grease a muffin mold, then put the melted cheese over the muffin holes in the bottom. Try to give the cheese the shape of the mold.
6. In a saucepan over medium heat, melt butter and add onions, stirring until golden and tender, then add garlic.
7. Pour the ground meat over the frying pan with the onion and the garlic, with the help of a wooden spoon, stir the meat to cook it, it will be ready when it is no longer pink. Proceed to remove excess fat.
8. Sprinkle the paprika, cumin, red pepper, salt, and pepper over the meat.
9. On the cheese baskets that you already cooked, pour the meat, stuffing it with meat, avocado, tomato, and sour cream.

BOMB BURGERS

This is a very simple recipe, which will allow you to savor the deliciousness of the meat, no need to leave the diet.

The ingredients are as follows:

- Butter or cooking spray. To add it to the muffin mold.
- One pound of ground beef.
- Half a spoonful of garlic powder, if you like, you can add more.
- Salt to taste.
- Pepper to taste.
- Two tablespoons of butter, divided into twenty pieces.
- Eight ounces of cheddar cheese, divided into twenty pieces.
- Leaves lettuce well washed.
- Tomatoes in thin slices.
- Mustard.

The preparation process is very simple:

1. Preheat oven to about 400°F.
2. The muffin mold, you can add the cooking spray, or butter, so that what we are going to put there does not get stuck.
3. Season the meat with the garlic powder, salt, and pepper.

4. Take a tablespoon of meat, and put it in the muffin molds, then press it into the bottom. Then place a piece of butter on top, and press again, in order to completely cover the bottom.
5. Place a piece of cheese on top of the meat and butter, in each muffin cup, obviously, and then press the cheese, so that it is completely covered by the meat.
6. Bake until the meat is well cooked.
7. Remove the meat from each cup of muffin, do it carefully, it is recommended to use a spatula.
8. Serve the meat with the lettuce, tomato, and mustard.

As you may have seen, these recipes for a healthy lunch are very simple and quick to make, you don't need to be a chef to be able to cook this, so you don't need so much knowledge to be able to make our lunches.

DINNERS

This is the last meal of our day; for this reason, this takes on a fundamental importance, and that is why it is important to make a good dinner.

BROCCOLI KETO SALAD

This is a very simple recipe, which will allow you to have a diet that will provide you with good nutrition and helps you to continue with your ketosis process.

The ingredients are as follows:

- Salt to taste.
- Three broccoli, chopped into small pieces.
- Half a cup of grated yellow cheddar cheese.
- A quarter onion, cut into very thin slices.
- One-quarter cup sliced toasted almonds.
- Three slices of bacon, well cooked and toasted, which you can place as you like in your salad, either shredded or chopped.
- Two spoonfuls of chives, fresh and freshly chopped.
- Two-thirds of a cup of mayonnaise.
- Three spoonfuls of cider vinegar.
- One tablespoon of Dijon mustard.
- Freshly ground black pepper.

The steps to cook our broccoli salad are as follows:

1. Boil a considerable amount of water in a pot, about six cups of water.
2. Prepare a large bowl of ice water.
3. Pour the broccoli over the pot of boiling water, cook until tender; this may take an interval of one or two minutes.
4. Remove and place in a bowl of ice water until cool.
5. Drain the broccoli flowers with a sieve.
6. In another bowl, place the mayonnaise, vinegar, mustard, pepper, and salt, and beat everything to combine the ingredients of the dressing, you must achieve a homogeneous mixture.
7. In the bowl where you are going to serve the salad, pour the broccoli, grated cheddar cheese, onion, toasted almonds, and bacon, stir and then pour over them the dressing, mix until all the ingredients are covered by the dressing.
8. Refrigerate until ready to serve.

As you could see, the recipe has no major complication and can be done in less than an hour, you don't need so much knowledge to make the salad, and you are feeding us very well.

CHICKEN WITH BACON, CHEESE AND RANCH DRESSING

This recipe is very simple, and very tasty, because who doesn't like chicken, or bacon, or melted cheese?. Well, this recipe brings the three things together, a perfect combination and full of flavor.

The ingredients are as follows:

- Four slices of thick bacon, a little wide.
- Four boneless chicken breasts. It's important that you don't have skin or anything, you could also use chicken Milanese.
- Salt to taste.
- Pepper to taste.
- Two spoonfuls of ranchero seasoning.
- A cup and a half of grated mozzarella cheese, you can also eat it with cheddar cheese, to give a more "American" touch.
- Chopped chives.

As you can see in the ingredients, nothing from the other world is asked for; we could even say that it is usual. Therefore, the preparation of this recipe does not come out very expensive, and besides, it does not consume much time, as you will see below:

1. In a frying pan over medium heat, proceed to cook the bacon, leaving them to fry on their own fat and leaving them crispy, turning them from time to time. This can last about eight minutes. It's best to do all of this on a large pan.
2. After the bacon is cooked, remove it to a plate and drain the remaining fat from each bacon, we recommend lining it with kitchen paper.
3. Drain the frying pan a little, throwing away a little of the fat that the bacon has thrown away, but we will not throw away all of it, but we will leave two or three spoonfuls of bacon oil.
4. Season your chicken with salt and pepper to taste.
5. Return the pan to medium heat, a little higher now, and proceed to put the chicken pieces, cook until the chicken is golden and ready, so that it is not raw, this can take about six minutes.
6. Lower the heat of your pan, and then add the powder or ranch dressing to the chicken, and finally, coat it with mozzarella or cheddar cheese.
7. Cover the frying pan with its lid, and wait for the cheese to melt, and bubbles begin to bubble out of it.
8. Chop the bacon in small pieces, and proceed to pour it over the cheese, do the same with the spring onion.

As you could see, this recipe is extremely simple and very tasty, as are most recipes that have a ketogenic food base. Therefore, we only have to tell you to keep practicing and make many more recipes to see that having this way of eating is not boring quite the opposite.

CHAPTER 17:
DRINKS AND DESSERTS

A positive aspect of the keto diet is the fact that we can continue to eat deliciously without so many limitations as our body goes into ketosis, cravings or that feeling of anxiety will disappear.

However, it is common that we have a craving from time to time and much more if before changing our eating habits we had the habit of eating sweets in large quantities, keto desserts will be our salvation and we can enjoy a good snack that satisfies our cravings without going out of line.

It has always been believed that healthy eating is a drastic and limiting change in our lives, and even has the belief that a snack has to be a fruit; if we look at this case, most of these fruits do not favor the keto diet, so we should look for other healthy alternatives that can help us.

Next, we will show you different types of desserts that we can make in the keto diet:

Keto Recipes That Do Dot Need to Be Cooked in the Oven

PEANUT BUTTER LINT FAT BOMBS

It is known that peanut butter is a delight if we add chocolate is a bomb explosion of flavors.

Ingredients:

- 1 cup of whipped cream
- 3 tablespoons natural peanut butter
- 100 grams of cream cheese
- 1 tablespoon vanilla
- 50 grams unsweetened chocolate (preferably dark chocolate)

Preparation mode:

1. In a bowl, add the whipped cream and stir until doubled in size.
2. In a separate bowl, mix the cream cheese with the natural peanut butter, chocolate, and vanilla; and mix until it looks like a soft, creamy lint.

3. Then we are going to unite all the ingredients in the same bowl, and we will be mixing slowly until they integrate correctly and are soft.
4. Additionally, we can add grated chocolate to decorate.

The best part is that this recipe only takes:

- Net carbohydrates: 2 g
- Calories: 140 g
- Fat: 14 g
- Proteins: 3 g

KETO CHEESECAKE

Ingredients:

- 120 g. cream cheese
- ¼ cup of sweetener
- ¼ cup thick whipped cream
- 2 tablespoons sour cream
- 60 grams of unsweetened pastry chocolate
- ½ cup whipped cream

Preparation:

1. With the help of a mixer, mix the cream cheese, sour cream, whipped cream, and sweetener.
2. Fill a cupcake mold with the mixture.
3. We take the refrigerator for 3 hours or the freezer for an hour and a half.
4. For the ganache:
5. Melt the chocolate pastry in the microwave.
6. Add the thick cream to whip.
7. Mix gently until it compacts, or you get a thick consistency.
8. Decorate to taste.

With this delicious recipe, we are enjoying a delicious combination of flavors without losing our line that has only:

- Carbohydrates: 3 g.
- Calories: 300 g.
- Fats: 35 g.
- Proteins: 5 g.

COCONUT BISCUITS

With Only 3 Ingredients (not baked)

- 3 cups finely grated coconut flakes.
- 1 cup coconut oil
- ½ cup of sweetener

Preparation:

1. In a bowl, mix the ingredients until we obtain a manipulable dough.
2. Form uniform balls and crush them into the shape of a biscuit.
3. Place each cookie 1 finger away in a tray with parchment paper.
4. Refrigerate until firm

This delicious recipe can be kept covered at room temperature for 7 days. If you only have the mixture, you can freeze it for up to 2 months.

Keto Recipes That Need an Oven for Preparation

CHOCOLATE CAKE OR KETOLATE CAKE

Ingredients:

For the cake:

- 1 1/2 cup almond flour
- 2/3 Tbsp sugar-free cocoa powder
- 3/4 cup coconut flour
- 2 tbsp. baking powder
- 2 tbsp. baking soda
- 500 grams of butter
- 1 cup sweetener
- 4 eggs
- 1 tablespoon vanilla
- 1 cup almond milk
- 1/3 cup of coffee

For frosting:

- 60 grams of cream cheese

- 250 grams of butter
- ½ cup sweetener (or to taste)
- 1/2 tbsp sugar-free cocoa powder
- 1/2 tbsp coconut flour
- 3/4 cup whipping cream

Preparation:

1. Preheat oven to 350 °.
2. Grease the mold where the cake is going to be baked.
3. In a large bowl, combine all dry ingredients
4. With the help of a blender, mix all the liquid ingredients.
5. Combine ingredients in one bowl
6. Bake for 30 minutes.
7. Preparation of the glaze: In a large bowl, with the help of a mixer mix the cream cheese and butter until a smooth mixture is formed, then gradually add the rest of the ingredients.
8. Decorate and serve

CHOCOLATE CHIP COOKIES

Ingredients:

- 2 eggs
- 250 grams melted butter
- 2 tablespoons whipping cream
- 2 teaspoons of vanilla
- 2 3/4 cup almond flour
- 1/4 cup granulated sugar keto-friendly
- 100 grams of dark chocolate in drops.

Preparation:

1. Preheat oven to 350 °.
2. In a large bowl mix the egg and butter
3. Then add the waiting cream and vanilla and mix until you add the dry ingredients.
4. Finally, add the chocolate sparks.
5. Form uniform balls and in a tray with parchment paper, place them with three fingers apart.

5. Bake for 15 minutes

What Beverages Other Than Water Can I Drink on the Keto Diet?

Among the most prominent are:

- Water infusions
- Hot or cold coffee
- Hot or cold tea
- Diet Sodas
- Smoothies keto

How to make Keto Infusions?

To make infusions is simpler than you can imagine. Besides that, they are very healthy giving us the capacity of up to 4 liters for preparation.

Strawberry and Cucumber Infusion

Ingredients:

- 500 g strawberries
- Cucumber slices
- 2 liters of water

OTHER TYPES OF KETO DRINKS

HOT CHOCOLATE

Ingredients:

- 2 spoonfuls. cocoa powder without sugar
- 2 1/2 teaspoons sweetener
- 1 1/4 cup water
- 1/4 cup heavy cream
- 1/4 teaspoon vanilla
- Whipped cream to taste, to decorate

Preparation:

1. In a saucepan, mix the cocoa, sweetener, and water on a medium-low heat until it dissolves correctly.

2. Increase heat to medium and add remaining ingredients, stirring constantly.
3. When it is hot enough, add the vanilla and serve in a cup.

KETO SMOOTHIE

Ingredients:

- Spinach
- coconut milk
- whey protein,
- Almonds
- Sweet potato starch
- psyllium seeds

Preparation:

Beat all ingredients in blender and serve.

STRAWBERRY MILKSHAKE

- 1 cup fresh strawberries
- 1 tsp vanilla
- 1 tbsp. coconut or almond oil
- 450ml coconut milk or Greek yogurt

Preparation:

Beat all ingredients in blender and serve.

CHIA SHAKE

Ingredients:

- 1 tablespoon of chia seeds (previously soaked in water for 10 minutes)
- ¼ cup coconut milk
- 1 avocado
- 1 tsp. cocoa beans
- 1 tsp. cocoa powder
- 1 tablespoon protein powder

- 1 tbsp. coconut oil

Preparation:

We blend all the ingredients so that all the ingredients are mixed correctly if you feel that it has become thick, you can add a little water.

Serve and enjoy

KETO GREEN MILKSHAKE

Ingredients:

- Cucumber
- Pineapple
- Kiwi
- Ginger
- Parsley
- 2 cups of water

Preparation:

Mix all the ingredients in a blender and serve.

Can I drink alcohol if I'm on the Keto Diet?

If we ingest alcohol while following the keto diet, our body will use this as a way to get energy before using the fat, but this could be contradictory because in the state of ketosis we look for our body to burn fat to get energy and thus lose weight, so the intake of alcohol could achieve effects contrary to those we seek to get.

CHAPTER 18: QUICK AND EASY DIFFERENT RECIPES

We know that time is money, but it still doesn't mean that just because we have a tight schedule in our daily routine, we can't afford to eat healthy. Below we will show you recipes for healthy and delicious foods that you can prepare in less than 20 minutes.

QUICK SALAD

Ingredients:

- 40 grams of green leaves (Lettuce or so)
- ½ sliced spring onion
- 1 carrot
- 1/2 avocado
- 20 gr. paprika
- 20 gr. tomatoes
- 120 grams of smoked salmon or chicken
- ¼ cup olive oil

Preparation:

1. First, we will chop all our ingredients to our preference
2. In a medium jar (or our taste) we will serve the green leaves at the bottom, followed by this we will add the rest of the ingredients, finally add the salmon or chicken and olive oil.
3. This way, we will have a quick and delicious lunch.

MUSHROOM TORTILLA

Ingredients:

- 4 eggs
- 25 g. butter
- 50 g. Grated cheese
- ¼ chopped yellow onion
- 4 mushrooms, sliced

- salt and pepper

Preparation:

1. In a bowl, mix the eggs with a fork until foamy, then add salt and pepper to taste.
2. In a frying pan over medium heat, fry the mushrooms together with the onion and butter until they are cooked.
3. Add the egg to the frying pan.
4. When the tortilla is half cooked, add the cheese
5. Using a spatula, fold the tortilla in half to give it consistency.
6. Remove from frying pan and serve.

SMOKED SALMON AND AVOCADO MEAL

Ingredients:

- 250 g smoked salmon
- 2 avocados
- salt and pepper

Preparation:

1. Chop the avocado into strips and place on a plate.
2. Serve the lounge
3. Add salt and pepper to taste.

CRISPY BACON

Ingredients

- 400 g bacon
- 1 cauliflower
- 50 grams of butter
- salt and pepper
- Oil

Preparation:

1. Chop the cauliflower into small pieces
2. Chop bacon into small pieces
3. Fry in a frying pan with butter until golden brown and crisp.

4. Serve with salt and pepper to taste.

CRABMEAT AND EGG

Ingredients

- 3 eggs
- 500 g canned crab meat
- 2 avocados
- ½ cup mayonnaise
- 1½ oz. spinach
- 2 tablespoons olive oil
- salt and pepper

Preparation:

1. we boil the eggs for about 10 minutes
2. We season the crab meat to your preference
3. Once the eggs are boiled, we'll remove the shell.
4. Serve on a plate with avocado chopped in strips
5. mix the mayonnaise with the crab meat
6. We'll sprinkle olive oil for seasoning.

CONCLUSION

Thank you for making it through to the end of Keto and intermittent fasting: Your Essential Guide for a Low-Carb diet to perfect mind-body balance, weight loss, with ketogenic Recipes to Maximize Your Health, we really hope it was informative and that you were able to learn all of the tools you needed to achieve your goal with the keto diet, whatever it was.

If you are reading this, it is because you made it through the book. And because of that, we want to congratulate you, since it means that you are completely decided and moving forward to change your body, your lifestyle, and most importantly, your mental and physical health. We really know that making such a change is not an easy task, and that is why we are really happy that you are so decided and interested in this diet.

Since the moment you bought this book, you became a winner. You became a champion. Not everyone is brave enough to dare to change in such a drastic way their nutrition and their feeding methods. Most people fear to fail, but what differences the normal people from the special people, the people that success, the people that get out of the comfort zone, is the discipline and perseverance towards reaching their goals.

Even if you are starting and find it really hard, or if you started but quitted, don't give up, keep pushing, keep trying and see amazing and unbelievable changes to start happening. This does not only applies to this diet but for everything in the life

Finally, if you found this book useful in any way, a review on Amazon is always appreciated!

Lightning Source UK Ltd.
Milton Keynes UK
UKHW051346050221
378303UK00002BA/6

9 781801 692533